Sex and Gender Differences
in Personal Relationships

Sex and Gender Differences in Personal Relationships

DANIEL J. CANARY
TARA M. EMMERS-SOMMER
with SANDRA FAULKNER

The Guilford Press
New York   London

© 1997 The Guilford Press
A Division of Guilford Publications, Inc.
72 Spring Street, New York, NY 10012
www.guilford.com

Printed in the United States of America

This book is printed on acid-free paper.

Last digit is print number: 9 8 7 6 5 4 3 2 1

Library of Congress Cataloging-in-Publication Data

Canary, Daniel J.
  Sex and gender differences in personal relationships /
Daniel J. Canary, Tara M. Emmers-Sommer with Sandra
Faulkner.
      p. cm. — (The Guilford series on personal
  relationships)
  Includes bibliographical references and index.
  ISBN 1-57230-256-9 —ISBN 1-57230-322-0 (pbk.)
  1. Interpersonal relations. 2. Interpersonal
communication. 3. Sex differences (Psychology)
I. Emmers-Sommer, Tara M. II. Faulkner, Sandra.
III. Title. IV. Series.
HM132.C343 1997
302—dc21   97-37290
                                                       CIP

Preface

> There are two types of people in this world—those
> who categorize people into one of two groups and
> those who do not.
>
> *—Popular paradox*

How men and women communicate in their personal relationships
has become a "hot" topic in both academic and popular discussions.
A common assumption stresses differences between men and women
that might explain problems between the sexes, which is conveyed
in generalizations that take the form "Women want this, whereas
men want that." Such views also suggest that people have only one
brand of each sex to choose from; that is, all men are alike and all
women resemble each other. In this book, we attempt to counter
the prevailing notion that differences between the sexes are constant
and reveal separate molds, and we present an alternative to categorical thinking about men and women in their personal relationships.

   As one might expect, we, the authors of this book, each have
background influences that compose our ideas about sex and gender
differences. For instance, Dan's influences include being born to a
dual-career couple, being raised by two independently minded
grandmothers from different cultures (one Mexican American and
one from New England), and (unfortunately) accepting early in his
research career the literature that presents men and women in
stereotypic ways. This last influence was a mistake of judgment,

v

although it resulted in publications in respected journals (e.g., Canary, Cunningham, & Cody, 1988; Canary & Spitzberg, 1987; Stafford & Canary, 1991). *Those studies surprisingly reported the opposite of the hypothesized sex differences,* which led Dan to a reevaluation of how men and women really do communicate in their close, personal relationships.

Tara was also born to a dual-career couple. Unlike the scope of "acceptable" and "unacceptable" behaviors prescribed by gender roles, however, the parental example in Tara's upbringing did not "fit" any particular role(s). Specifically, both her parents worked, both did household chores, both took responsibility for the finances, both took care of the yard, and both shared child care responsibilities. Outside of the home, however, Tara heard what girls and boys, men and women "should" do. Such experiences included being told to "act ladylike" as a young child; being advised from a high school teacher upon learning of her interest in the law, "You don't look like a lawyer, but you look like you'd marry one"; and recently reading a real estate advertisement that touted a home as being "near the mall" for the mothers and "near the interstate" for fathers commuting into work. It is unfortunate—but evident—that stereotypes remain and women especially appear to be professionally handicapped by them.

One relevant influence is the recent popular portrayal of men and women. In 1990, Deborah Tannen published her widely accepted quasi-academic book, *You Just Don't Understand,* wherein men and women were cast as though they come from different cultures. Academics and lay people alike read Tannen's accounts of various "composite" couples and appreciated the nuance that Tannen offered. In addition, the two-cultures approach offered an alternative, though not necessarily an opposite point of view, to the dominance perspective that was popular in the 1970s and 1980s. Then John Gray (1992) exaggerated sex differences even further with the analogy that men are from Mars and women are from Venus, a thought that was inspired by the film *E.T.* (Gleick, 1997). The "nonfiction" portrayals by Tannen and Gray of men's and women's communication remained best sellers for years.

As we show in this book, most of the research does *not* support the view that men and women come from separate cultures, let alone separate worlds. Long-presumed differences in men's and women's interpersonal behavior simply do not reflect in the empirical research literature. Sex differences do not emerge because many researchers (like lay individuals) rely on traditional sex stereotypes when constructing the difference argument (i.e., men are instrumental, assertive, insensitive, and dominant, whereas women are communal, passive, sensitive, and subordinate), and the research shows that sex stereotypes poorly predict interpersonal communication behaviors.

Indeed, research suggests far more similarity than differences in men's and women's communication. For example, Canary and Hause (1993) reviewed 15 meta-analyses (representing some 1,200 studies) regarding sex differences in social behavior and found that about only 1% of the variance in people's social behavior derives from sex differences. Likewise, in the area of organizational communication, Wilkins and Andersen's (1991) meta-analysis (which was missed by Canary & Hause) found only one-half of 1% variance in behavior that was due to sex differences. According to these objective summaries, men and women are much more similar than different. If men and women do originate from different cultures or worlds, they at least speak the same language about 99% of the time.

Yet no one can deny that men and women are different. The issue is to provide some account of sex or gender that provides more insights than stereotypes can offer. Recently, scholars in psychology, communication, sociology, and related fields have offered theoretical models regarding men's and women's interaction in general that do not rely on stereotypic beliefs (e.g., Deaux & Major, 1987). In this book, we have pursued the specific objective of uncovering sex differences in *personal relationships*.

Research on sex differences too often has relied on strangers or acquaintances or hypothetical situations ("Imagine you are having a fight with your partner: What would you say?"). Predictably, much of the research also relies on college students, freshly emerged from adolescence and still trying to figure out for themselves how men and women communicate. Drawing inferences from such data appears to us as problematic at best. Accordingly, we attempted to stress the literature that focuses on people in close relationships, nonstudents in addition to students.

The research literature suggests a need to provide a context of men's and women's emotional reactions—how men and women might experience and express their responses to each other. Thus, we discuss emotional reactions. In addition, the literature indicates that two fundamental dimensions exist whereby people define their relationships. These dimensions are *intimacy* and *control*. Accordingly, we also review in two chapters the research on how men and women communicate intimacy and control in their personal relationships. Again, this literature shows that men and women communicate intimacy and control in more interesting ways than those suggested by sex stereotypes.

Beyond the sex difference issue—how one's biological sex affects one's behavior—we wanted also to underscore differences due to one's *gender*—the social–psychological–cultural manifestations of one's sex role identity. In our view, people create their gender in their various activities with each other. Especially in personal relationships, where normative expectations give way to relational expectations that are implicitly or explicitly negotiated between partners, people can and do create gender.

Our hope is to represent men and women sharing spheres cocreated through communication and inhabiting spheres with permeable boundaries. As we articulate in this book, a primary sphere of people's activity involves the division of household labor. Within that sphere, men and women have developed a range of communication strategies that directly or indirectly make statements like, "Because this task does not fall within the purview of being a man/woman, you should do it" and "I am more competent at this, so I will do it." A secondary sphere of activity is how men and women spend their leisure time—together and separately. These activities, and the communication that establishes and maintains them, provide the stage for creating gender in personal relationships.

How scholars and lay people conceptualize sex and/or gender differences varies radically. Accordingly, we do not anticipate widespread agreement with the points we make. We do hope for continued discussion about how men and women do, in fact, communicate and create expectations.

Many people still rely on stereotypes for their judgments on the issue of sex differences. But such a reliance on stereotypes only serves to perpetuate them among students and lay persons. In our view, the perpetuation of stereotypes constitutes the most disheartening outcome of books that distort and emphasize sex differences. If people come to believe that they are from separate cultures or worlds and that their social behavior is cast from separate molds, then they may never accept the idea that they can create their own gendered identities. As a result, advances in social, political, and economic equity might be handicapped by outdated notions of what men and women are capable of doing. This book provides one in a series of academic attempts to correct an antiquated, unfair portrayal of women and men. Many people still measure a man by his career advancement and intelligence and a woman by her looks and spending habits. In light of widespread acceptance of such notions, our goal is to examine men and women in close relationships without assuming one sex is attracted to the mall, and the other a "cave" (Gray, 1992).

A critically important influence on us are the people who have provided help at various stages of this project. At the top of this list is Steve Duck, editor of The Guilford Series on Personal Relationships. Steve Duck continues to advance the study of personal relationships in many ways, and he indeed provided insightful, coherent, and concrete advice to us about previous drafts. We owe Steve a debt of gratitude. In addition, several colleagues reviewed our book and offered us very helpful comments: Peter Andersen, San Diego State University; Kathryn Dindia, University of Wisconsin–Milwaukee; and Sandra Ragan, University of Oklahoma. The feedback that they provided markedly improved our book. Any flaws remaining in the present text are the result of our own decisions, not of any of these scholars.

We must mention the contribution of Sandra Faulkner (Penn State University), who as a research assistant read the manuscript, double-checked references, offered critical comments, and proposed additions we had not considered. Sandra's influence revived the project during a hot, muggy summer, and so we requested that she contribute to it. Her contribution can be detected in the ways we frame several of the ideas and in approximately 15 pages of original material. However, Sandra's views about feminist theory, women's health, and interpersonal interaction are much more extensive than this book can possibly indicate.

Several other individuals who contributed at various stages of writing deserve mention. The first is Peter Wissoker, the editor who patiently managed the book from proposal to postmark. Peter encouraged us to generate a strong theoretical statement in addition to a review of scholarly work. At first we were daunted by the suggestion; now we are very glad that he expressed his editor's intuition. Jim McCroskey (West Virginia University) also encouraged us to take a closer look at sex differences in communicative behavior, and we appreciate his advice. In addition, we wish to thank Charlene "Charlie" Dellinger. Charlie advised us years ago to explore the division of household labor ("You *must* read Hochschild's book"), and we are certainly glad she was clear in offering this advice and in writing an intriguing dissertation (School of Interpersonal Communication, Ohio University). Dennis Gouran (Penn State University) generously provided research assistants. Andy Gustafson (Penn State University) found and photocopied articles on sex differences as part of his research assistantship (RA). Andy was an assiduous RA, and he often returned with much more information than was requested of him.

Finally, we want to thank the people at The Guilford Press for their fine efforts. In addition to Peter Wissoker, we are grateful for the work of William Meyer, April Heck, and Kimberley Windbiel, who were very thorough and thoughtful. Additionally, we thank Robert Egert for his provocative book cover. We are most appreciative for the combined efforts of this excellent group of people.

Contents

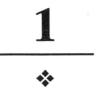

1

❖

Moving Beyond Stereotypes

DO MEN AND WOMEN INHABIT DIFFERENT WORLDS?

John Gray's *Men Are from Mars, Women Are from Venus* (1992) has sold over 6 million copies—more than any other nonfiction hardcover book (Gleick, 1997, p. 69). Gray argues that men and women are so entirely different that it appears they come from different planets. And these planets have alternative meanings for the same language. But somewhere along the way, we have forgotten that men and women originated in different worlds and that we need an interpreter (John Gray?) to help us understand each other. This analogy not only provides the foundation for Gray's portrayal of personal relationships between men and women, it also serves as the premise for the entire book (and several other books Gray has written). Gray's success in using this figurative analogy as a premise for understanding men and women cannot be denied in a social or monetary sense—Gray enjoys thousands of loyal followers and has earned approximately $18 million from book sales alone (i.e., not counting money he gets from seminars [$35, 000 per engagement], Mars and Venus Counseling Centers, or multimedia [videos, CDs, etc.]; Gleick, 1997).

Of course, Gray's figurative analogy presents a polarized view of men and women communicating with each other. For example, consider the following passage about how one sex difference hurts relationships:

> Women generally do not understand how Martians [men] cope with stress. They expect men to open up and talk about all their problems the way Venusians [women] do. When a man is stuck in his cave, a woman resents his not being more open. She feels hurt when he turns on the news or goes outside to play some basketball and ignores her.
>
> To expect a man who is in his cave instantly to become open, responsive, and loving is as unrealistic as expecting a woman who is upset immediately to calm down and make complete sense. It is a mistake to expect a man to always be in touch with his loving feelings just as it is a mistake to expect a woman's feelings to always be rational and logical. (p. 33)

To the extent one accepts the premise that men and women are so different they seem to come from different social and psychological worlds, Gray's many prescriptions regarding communication make sense. However, to the extent one finds the premise grossly exaggerated (and it is), then such a polarizing and stereotypic presentation of men and women appears fictional and offensive (see Crawford, 1995, for other examples regarding Gray's extreme position).

Although polarized portrayals of men and women may be entertaining (see also Tannen, 1990), one must wonder at their effect on people's understanding of sex and gender roles and how men and women *should* act in their close relationships. Geis (1993), for example, has provided evidence that at a general social level stereotypes act as value-laden, self-fulfilling prophecies. In other words, stereotypes about men and women become standards for behavior. Moreover, people have a tendency to create bipolar constructs, and thereby they essentialize the "male" and "female" qualities (Thorne, 1990). The question then is whether such polarized views function for the social good, for scientific purposes, or whether they have little social or scientific payoff.

Putnam (1982) argued that nothing can be gained by polarizing men and women through reliance on stereotypes. More specifically, she pointed out that understanding sex/gender differences in social interaction behavior requires more than an affirmation of sex stereotypes that portray women as communal (i.e., primarily concerned with relational welfare) and men as instrumental (i.e., primarily concerned with task-related resources) . She described the landscape of scientific theory on the issue as "barren," largely due to the polarizations of men and women that reside in traditional stereotypes.

Of course, many scholars have invested considerable effort in delineating the structure and content of sex stereotypes (e.g., Eagly & Steffen, 1984). Deaux and Lewis (1984) reported that the stereotypical man is instrumental, assertive, competitive, dynamic, and task-competent, whereas the stereotypical woman is kind, nurturing, sensitive, relationally oriented, and expressive. These authors found that their participants rely on such labels until they learn more specific information about one another, as partners do in close relationships.

Stereotypes can offer a means to explain sex and gender differences on at least two levels: (1) as a way to predict men's and women's behavioral differences; and (2) as a way that people establish baselines for expectations about other people's behavior. In the former case, researchers adopt sex role stereotypes to construct their own concepts and measures (e.g., Bem, 1974); in the latter case, researchers hold that participants rely on stereotypes to know how to behave or to judge behavior (e.g., Geis, 1993).

The problem does not reside in the theoretical construction and explanation of the understanding of the nature and function of stereotypes in interaction behavior; rather, the problem arises when researchers uncritically—and perhaps without realizing they do so—adopt stereotypes as a means for scientifically explaining and predicting sex and gender differences. Adopting stereotypic thinking represents a rather simple solution to the sex difference issues, although as a solution it is inadequate because people do not reliably conform in their interaction behavior to conventional sex stereotypes (Aries, 1996). Although we concur with Deaux (1984) and others who claim that sex stereotypes are pervasive, we also contend that they appear baldly essentializing in their portrayals of men's and women's behavior. In particular, we contend that stereotypes do not adequately or accurately represent men's and women's interactions in personal relationships.

We acknowledge that men and women sometimes differ in their interaction behavior and they sometimes rely on stereotypes as guidelines for interaction behavior (Deaux & Major, 1987). However, such stereotypes present an outdated view of men and women that distorts scientific understandings of male and female interaction, *especially in the context of personal relationships.* If one holds than men are from Mars and women are from Venus, then it follows that Earth provides no home for either sex.

INVESTIGATING SEX AND GENDER DIFFERENCES IN PERSONAL RELATIONSHIPS

This book relies on several assumptions and seeks to advance a few objectives. First, we wish to show that stereotypic knowledge about men and women fails to predict interaction in close involvements. Although we see this task as a small hurdle, we find it remarkable that so much research on sex/gender differences still relies on stereotypic understandings of men and women. Although we agree that stereotypes provide information about the nature and function of social categories, we do not believe that they constitute a powerful predictor or indicator of interaction in close relationships. We will take up this first objective shortly.

Second, we recognize the potential for a greater understanding of actual interaction behavior. We hope to provide a balanced view (i.e., locating sex/gender differences as well as similarities), although we acknowledge that our own personal schemata and biases have inevitably filtered our understanding of the literature. In the past, researchers have sought to explain sex and gender differences without an eye toward understanding the similarities. The result was a bipolar, essentialized picture of men and women. More current efforts, however, appear to stress contexts and activities that men and women share as well as those that reveal differences (e.g., Aries, 1996). We view this book as part of this current trend to balance discussions about sex/gender differences with sex/gender similarities.

Finally, our efforts will assess, however indirectly, the equality as well as inequality that exist between men and women in personal relationships. The nature of equality carries with it social, political, and critical overtones. We need to be clear that we have no social or critical cause per se, although the research literature might indicate several areas where inequality exists and can be repaired. We do not, however, presume that either men or women separately own the burden of repairing inequality. In our view, gender is a relational construct that two people create through interaction with each other.

We begin our analysis by defining *sex* and *gender.* Then we address the fundamental issue of whether or not the research supports a presumption of sex/gender differences or sex/gender similarities.

Defining Sex and Gender

Defining terms is an important obligation because definitions establish the boundaries of a phenomenon and indicate one's under-standing of it. We have considered several issues in the debate over the definition of the terms *sex* and *gender.* For instance, some scholars hold that gender is partially composed of one's biological sex, but that gender also entails "the psychological, social, and cultural features and characteristics strongly associated with the biological categories of male and female" (Gilbert, 1993, p. 11). Likewise, Moore (1994) has argued that the construct of sex entails both a reference to objective differences in the genetic/biological composi-tion of men and women and to people's beliefs accompanying the term "sex"; gender refers to the cultural understandings and expla-nations that people have for sex. Accordingly, "sex" is partially socially constructed, is sometimes conflated with *sexuality,* and connotes sexual intercourse. In the scholarly debate about the term "gender," some argue that gender refers to cultural differences between men and women, whereas others argue that gender is a grammatical device (as in "masculine" nouns), and still others argue that gender refers exclusively to "women" and women's attitudes and behaviors (Scott, 1996).

Despite the definitional debates on the topic, which can appear quite nuanced, we opt for a clear distinction. More precisely, we adopt the advice set forth in the *Journal of Social and Personal Relationships* (*JSPR*) and define *sex* as the biological distinctions between men and women and *gender* as the social, psychological, and cultural differentiations between men and women (see also Deaux, 1985). This convention allows us to be clear about our terms, and this distinction appears to be gaining support among those who define *sex* versus *gender*. Moreover, we consider *JSPR* to be the most important scholarly journal promoting the study of personal relationships (with importance defined in terms of longevity, circulation, impact, quantity of citations, and quality of research).

By extension, studies that examine social differences between men and women as separate biological categories provide information about *sex differences,* whereas studies that rely on socially constructed notions of male and female refer to *gender differences* (Deaux, 1985). In addition, one's "sex role identity" refers to instances wherein one's self-concept is linked to biological differences (e.g., "motherhood"), whereas "gender role identity" refers to the degree to which one's self-concept connects to psychological dimensions for understanding men and women as social, goal-directed beings (e.g., "as a nurturing parent"; Eagly, 1987). Likewise, "sex roles" refer to expectations thought to derive naturally from one's biological sex, whereas "gender roles" pertain to expectations that psychologically and socially define the enactment of gender.

We attempt to remain consistent in our own use of these terms. In addition, we refer to sex *and* gender or *sex/gender* when we discuss both constructs (e.g., as a general domain of inquiry). We also replace terms used by other authors in quotes in order to maintain consistency in meaning, and we do so only when one term clearly is implied over the other. This most often meant replacing "gender" with "sex," to indicate differences between men and women as genetically separate groups. However, we did not replace terms when one term was not clearly used as we have defined these terms above.

Our view of the relationship between sex and gender is more fully articulated in Chapter 6. At this point, however, we want to stress that we consider *gender* to be constructed in the activities of men and women, the most primary activity being social interaction; and one's genetic/biological *sex* implicitly influences the social construction of gender. As Thompson and Walker (1989) noted,

"Gender is something evoked, created, and sustained day-by-day through interaction among family members" (p. 865). Similarly, Hare-Mustin and Marecek (1988) pointed out, "Constructing gender is a process, not an answer" (p. 462). Likewise, Rakow (1986) claimed that "gender is both something we do and something we think with, both a set of social practices and a system of cultural meanings" (p. 21).

Assessing the Presumption of Differences

One does not need supporting research to claim that sex differences exist. Men and women obviously differ. Men's genetic code differs from women's, men have historically enjoyed greater sociopolitical power and status, and women have been conferred greater prestige in relationship matters. Yet precisely *how* men and women differ in their personal relationships remains quite a mystery, especially in comparison to sex differences on display in physical and sociopolitical realms of behavior. Sex and gender differences in personal relationships emerge in minute interaction behaviors, often in private contexts, and within different subcultures that defy sweeping, categorical generalizations about men's and women's behaviors in "society at large."

The issue of whether or not pervasive sex/gender differences exist in personal relationships is addressed variously and often inferred from research involving acquaintances or strangers. For example, Henley (1977) focused on how women suffer power deficits in the context of cross-sex interaction, arguing that men's greater occupational status affords them more power and freedom in several behavioral categories: space (e.g., women use less space in interactions with men), time (e.g., women wait on men), environment (e.g., women have less freedom to arrange their environment), language (e.g., men talk longer), demeanor (e.g., men act more relaxed), touch (men can, women cannot), eye contact (men stare, have higher visual dominance scores), and facial expression (e.g., women must offer a pleasant smile). Henley's review strongly supported the contention that men consistently dominate women through communication behavior.

More recently, scholars in the fields of communication, psychology, and family studies (among others) have begun to doubt findings regarding sex/gender differences that reflect the traditional women-as-communal and men-as-instrumental categories (e.g., various views by authors in Canary & Dindia, in press). Ragan (1989) observed that the study of sex differences in communication presents no single consistent finding. In a noteworthy paper, Duck and Wright (1993) reversed their own earlier interpretations of two sets of data to conclude that, within the sexes, the friendships of men and women were more similar than different: "Within sexes, characteristics that are important in friendship do not fit readily into expressive vs. instrumental categories for either women or men. That is, according to our factor analyses, expressive and instrumental characteristics are about equally prominent aspects of a strong friendship for both women and men" (p. 724). Analyzing the research on group interaction using Interaction Process Analysis (IPA), Aries (1996) also reversed an earlier claim she made that supported the stereotype of men as instrumental and women as communal:

> Many studies using IPA or a variant of the 12 categories have supported the original findings by Strodbeck and Mann [1956] that in groups men show more task behavior and women more social–emotional behavior. While the case has been made that men are instrumental and women expressive, a closer examination of these studies suggests that this stereotyped description of men and women is an exaggeration of the data, that the differences are small to moderate in magnitude, and that role differentiation along instrumental–expressive lines by males and females does not appear consistently in all group situations. (p. 27)

Aries (1996) proceeded to review, in detail, interaction differences between men and women in a variety of behavioral domains (i.e., self-disclosure, leadership behaviors, interruptions, conversational management, etc.), and she concluded, "I have gone back through the research literature to demonstrate that the data reveal similarities between men and women to be far greater than the differences, and that knowledge about a person's [sex] will give us little ability to accurately predict how a person will behave in many situations" (p. 189).

In addition, meta-analyses (i.e., statistical summaries of research) have revealed that sex differences account for little variance in social interaction behavior. As an illustration, Wilkins and Andersen (1991) examined the studies on sex differences in communication behavior observed within organizations. Wilkins and Andersen found that only 0.5% of communication behavior could be accounted for by one's sex. Summaries of meta-analyses relevant to interaction behavior reveal that sex differences appear to be quite small. Canary and Hause (1993), for example, reviewed 15 meta-analyses that revealed an average sex effect that accounted for only about 1% of variation in people's communication-relevant behavior (average $d = .23$). In other words, men and women respond in a similar manner 99% of the time. Table 1.1 reports the meta-analyses summarized by Canary and Hause.

On the other hand, Hall's (1984) exhaustive study of nonverbal behavior indicated that nonverbal communication qualifies as one area in which sex differences remain robust. Table 1.2 reports a summary of Hall's findings that includes adults (and which also can include children). Additionally, Hall (in press) reviewed studies in psychology in general, and nonverbal behavior in particular, and reported that sex differences in the specific areas of smiling and nonverbal sensitivity "are relatively large" (i.e., r's range from .25 to .30). Hall concluded that sex differences for nonverbal behavior appear larger than sex differences in other domains of psychology. However, Dindia (J. T. Wood & Dindia, in press) combined the findings from Canary and Hause with those reported by Hall, and found that the average weighted effect size due to sex differences remained at 1–2% of the variance. At a minimum, these summaries of meta-analyses suggest that wide variation exists even in the interpretation of relatively "objective" summaries of sex differences.[1]

In a recent issue of *American Psychologist,* researchers debated the issue of how large sex differences appear to be and how to interpret effect sizes involving sex differences. Eagly (1995) argued that although effect sizes due to sex differences appear small to moderate, sex differences nevertheless account for as much of the variance as one would expect from any psychological construct. Eagly urged readers to consider the relative "benchmarks" of similar research when examining sex differences. On the other hand, Hyde and Plant (1995) argued that sex differences as a rule appear to be small, and they report that 25% of sex difference research reveals a "close to zero" effect, 35% of the research shows a small effect, and 13% of

TABLE 1.1. Summary of 15 Meta-Analyses

Author(s)	No. of studies (No. of subjects)	Results	d
Dindia & Allen (1992)	205 (N = 23,702)	Women disclose more	.18
Eagly & Carli (1981)	148: 61 persuasion studies;	Women are more influenceable	.16
	64 conformity studies with pressure;	Women conform more • with pressure	.32
	23 conformity studies without pressure (Mdn N's = 166.00; 75.50; 81.13)	• without pressure	.28
Eagly & Crowley (1986)	182 (Mdn N = 159.88)	Men help more	.34
Eagly & Johnson (1990)	144 (Mdn N = 88)	Women lead more	.03
Eagly & Karau (1991)	75 (Mdn N = 80)	Men emerge more as leaders in • task measures	.41
		• unspecified measures	.29
		Women emerge more as leaders in • social measures	.18
Eagly, Makhijani, & Klonsky (1992)	147 (Mdn obs = 80)	Female leaders are evaluated less favorably	.05
Eagly & Steffen (1986)	81 (Mdn N = 84.50)	Men are more aggressive	.40
		Men receive more aggression	.32
Hyde & Linn (1988)	165	Women are more verbally skilled	.11
Swim, Borgida, Maruyama, & Meyers (1989)	106 (N = 21,379)	Women are judged as more competent	.08
Wood (1987)	52 (Mdn N = 59.6)	Men outperform women in groups	.38

Note. d, weighted mean difference in standard deviation units. Unreported moderators and interactions were significant at $p < .05$. Adapted from Canary and Hause (1993, p. 131). Copyright 1993 by Eastern Communication Association. Adapted by permission.

TABLE 1.2. Hall's Analysis of Sex Differences in Nonverbal Behavior

Nonverbal behavior	No. of studies	Association	r^2
Decoding skill	64	.21	.04
Face recognition	12	.17	.03
Expression skill	35	.25	.06
Facial expressiveness	5	.45	.20
Social smiling	15	.30	.09
Gazing	30	.32	.10
Receipt of gaze	6	.31	.10
Distance of approach			
To others (naturalistic)	17	−.27	.07
By others (naturalistic)	9	−.43	.18
Body movement/position			
Restlessness	6	−.34	.12
Expansiveness	6	−.46	.21
Involvement	7	.16	.03
Expressiveness	7	.28	.08
Self-consciousness	5	.22	.05
Vocal behavior			
Speech errors	6	−.33	.11
Filled pauses	6	−.51	.26
Total speech	12	−.05	.00

Note. The association refers to *r*, where positive values indicate higher values on the behavior by females. (Squaring the measure of association reveals the effect due to sex.) Studies within the categories of expression skill and body movement are not independent. Adapted from Hall (1984, p. 142). Copyright 1984 by Johns Hopkins University Press. Adapted by permission.

the studies are in the large or extremely large effect size categories. Hyde and Plant interpreted these data as showing more similarity than difference between men and women in terms of their psychological construction.

Factors Affecting the Presumption of Differences

Several factors can help explain why scholars cannot agree on whether sex differences account for substantial or negligible portions of social behavior. First, at a theoretical level, some scholars presume that one's biological sex provides a primary means for understanding social interaction, whereas others adopt a more skeptical posture in presuming that no differences exist until empirically demonstrated otherwise. Hare-Mustin and Marecek (1988) observed that those who presume sex differences in behavior suffer from "alpha bias," or "the exaggeration of differences" (p. 457). Hare-Mustin and Marecek noted that many approaches to examining sex difference suffer from alpha bias, including the perspectives of Bacon, Freud, and Parsons, as well as that of cultural feminism. That is, these and other scholars presume that women and men are essentially different. On the other hand, researchers who adopt a "beta bias" presume that no differences between men and women exist. According to Hare-Mustin and Marecek (1988), family systems theorists who emphasize age over sex, for example, may miss effects that have to do with the sex difference between fathers and mothers. In short, one's initial expectation for difference partially determines how one frames the sex and gender difference issue and how one interprets both quantitative and qualitative data on sex differences. More scholars appear to have alpha than beta biases; that is, they operate from the presumption that differences exist until they are proven not to exist (Bem, 1993; Hare-Mustin & Marecek, 1988; cf. Eagly, 1995).

Second, and related to the observation that most researchers presume sex and gender differences, null hypotheses excite very few people (and we cannot be too sure about those few who are excited by them). As a rule, people do not pay millions of dollars for books about sameness, and researchers do not joyfully report results that support null hypotheses. Science, after all, is the study of variance.

Many of the studies reporting differences in fact overlook similarities that outweigh the differences.[2] Differences appear informative, interesting, and meaningful in terms of explaining variance, so researchers often emphasize these in interpreting findings and explain away the similarities; or they manage the data to emphasize differences (e.g., by establishing a ceiling on the number of hours men work outside the home to 40 per week), or they do not *test* for sex differences but eyeball the data and presume large differences. As Crawford (1995) indicated, "The template provided speech stereotypes has sometimes led to what might be called empiricist revisionism, in which results counter to received beliefs about women's [versus men's] speech are reinterpreted to fit" (p. 30).

For example, Wright (in press) reviewed data pertaining to men's and women's friendships and found that men and women appear more similar than different in terms of their instrumentality, whereas sex differences are larger in terms of communality. Yet, researchers have consistently argued fallaciously and without the appropriate statistical analysis that women's relationships are communal and men's are instrumental (Wright, in press). The point is that sex differences are not absolute as much as they are gradual and complex (Deaux, 1984). Allowing that similarities between men and women exist should help us understand more precisely where sex/gender differences occur.

A third influence on one's research arises from one's own social contacts. For instance, Fitzpatrick (1988a) has shown that sex differences appear more marked in "Traditional" couples than in "Independent" couples. According to Fitzpatrick, Traditional couples adopt a conventional ideology concerning how men and women should behave; women take men's last names during marriage, for example. Independent couples do not adhere to conventional norms regarding gender roles; they might argue about whose turn it is to cook or clean, for instance. Fitzpatrick argued that our understanding of marriage emerges from our families of origin in the form of schemas. Accordingly, people (including researchers) raised in Traditional households will likely adopt conventional gender roles, and those raised in Independent households will likely adopt egalitarian gender roles. Of course, people rely on sources—including their own experiences—other than their family of origin, and these other sources presumably can mass in an additive manner to construct alternative prototypes of what it means to be a man and a woman, a male and female friend, a brother and a sister, a husband and a wife.

Fourth, researchers are like most people—they value and protect their ideological preferences, some of which predispose them to "spin" the sex/gender difference debate in a particular way. Deaux (1985) said, "The interface of ideology with the scientific enterprise, long a topic of debate for social science research in general, supplies a tension that pervades the area [of sex differences in psychology]. What one may wish as a feminist is not necessarily what one sees as a scientist" (p. 74). Similarly, Tannen (1994) stated, "Entering the arena of research on gender is like stepping into a maelstrom. What it means to be female or male, what it's like to talk to someone of the other (or the same) [sex], are questions whose answers touch people where they live, and when a nerve is touched, people howl" (p. 3).

Current stereotypes of men and women imply a cultural value regarding men and women (Geis, 1993; J. J. Wood, 1993). Stereotypes and the values attached to them often appear to guide researchers' interpretations of findings (whether they support sex similarity or sex difference). Of course, before the feminist critique, much theoretical research presumed an *androcentric* posture (i.e., "man" provided a valid frame of reference for judging behavior of men and women; Bem, 1993).

In a related vein, people do not appear to know how to interpret the entire issue of sex and gender differences within a feminist ideology. For example, Eagly (1995) claimed that "empirical feminists" prefer to read about sex similarities, rather than differences. However, Hyde and Plant (1995) noted that although some feminists are "minimalists" who claim that few if any differences exist between men and women, other feminists are "maximalists" who seek to point out differences between the sexes. We concur with Marecek's (1995) comment on this issue: "From my vantage point, there is little sign of anything resembling a monolithic feminist agenda. Instead, there is a profusion of diverging goals, interests, and visions put forward by different groups of women. This profusion is so great that some feel they can speak only of feminisms, not feminism" (p. 163).

In short, once a person has adopted a belief regarding gendered behavior, values associated with stereotypes, and/or an ideological framework for explaining men and women, one cannot easily dismiss those points of reference simply because of some anomalous findings that fall outside of one's belief system (Crawford, 1995). Scholars place at stake their personal experiences and ideological values when they read, research, and discuss sex differences, and such values are nearly impossible to discard. For example, in the preface of her book, Henley (1977) boldly presented her purpose: "This book is . . . especially for women who have been oppressed by power because of their sex and who are more affected by body politics than men are" (p. vii). It is no surprise to us that Henley's review documented how men use nonverbal cues to dominate women.

Finally, as many experts on the topic note (e.g., Aries, in press; Deaux, 1985; Eagly, 1987), sex differences reveal few consistent main effects apart from other contextual factors. Sex differences emerge in different ways depending on other characteristics of the situation, the task at hand, the partner, and other moderating variables. Accordingly, obtaining a clear view of sex differences requires an examination of the context wherein the interaction occurs. Dismissing the moderating factors in hopes of finding "pure" sex differences may actually prevent us from finding systematic variance due to sex. In other words, assuming monolithic and powerful main effects due to one's biological sex or psychological gender only impedes understanding of how people relate to each other in close involvements. At this juncture, we elaborate on this point more by delineating several issues that researchers and readers alike must somehow consider when examining sex differences in close, personal relationships.

A FLOWCHART MODEL PREDICTING STEREOTYPIC INTERACTION BEHAVIOR

We believe that sex differences exist, but the manner in which they emerge in interaction behavior between partners remains opaque. As indicated above, the primary culprit for the fuzzy picture appears to be researchers' reliance on and perpetuation of exaggerated, "main effect" polarization arising from stereotypes (see also Aries, 1996; Putnam, 1982; Ragan, 1989). If we consider various models for sex-linked behavior (i.e., that within-group differences exist for men and women), and if we allow for various countervailing influences on one's communication behavior, then we should find as invalid studies presuming that stereotypes are powerful influences. Figure 1.1 presents what researchers and readers need to address when presupposing stereotypic behavior.

The model we offer in Figure 1.1 indicates how sex-relevant beliefs affect interaction (see also Deaux & Major, 1987). The flowchart in Figure 1.1 offers five questions that people should consider regarding behavior between close relationship partners (e.g., self-disclosure, touch, conflict). Our objective in this exercise is to show some of the pitfalls contained in the presumption of stereotypic sex differences in personal relationships. We assume that the mediating factors listed in Figure 1.1 are most often significant in personal relationships. In addition, we assume that during interaction two people are communicating, although this model might apply to other contexts (e.g., small groups, organizations). Finally, we focus on the sex-relevant behaviors of one person at a time (i.e., the *actor*), which reflects other researchers' view of sex as an individual, structural variable. The same questions addressed at the dyadic level would double and become more difficult to answer. Nevertheless, the search for stereotypic sex differences progresses as one answers each of the following questions:

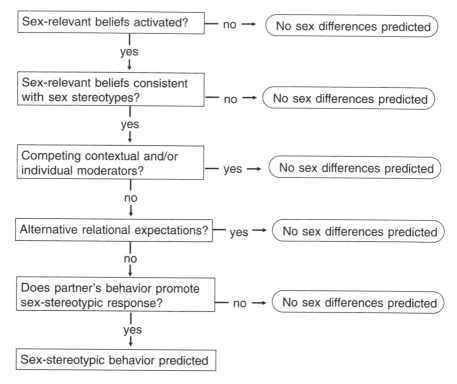

FIGURE 1.1. Model predicting sex-stereotypic interaction behaviors.

1. *Are the actor's sex-relevant beliefs activated?* By *activation* we refer to any context-specific stimulus that elicits a sex-relevant schema, script, or prototype. Deaux and Major (1990) noted the following:

> Both parties in an interaction can influence the likelihood of gender schemata being activated. Specific features of a person's appearance can trigger a subset of gender beliefs in the mind of the observer, for example, shifting the expectancies from those associated with women and men in general to those linked to more particular subtypes. A woman with a briefcase elicits different associations for most people than does a woman in an apron and housedress. (p. 96)

An important, though often presumed, condition concerns whether or not interaction parties' sex-relevant beliefs are activated. In some cases, the briefcase (or housedress) may not elicit a person's schemata for sex-relevant responses. If routine stimuli fail to generate one's sex-relevant beliefs, then the answer to the first question is "no, sex relevant beliefs are not activated in this situation," and one's search for stereotypically defined sex differences concludes. If the answer is "yes," then one must proceed to address the next question.

2. *Do the actor's sex-relevant beliefs conform to the conventional stereotype?* People hold various beliefs about men and women, and some of these beliefs reflect stereotypes (Bem, 1981). According to Bem's gender schema theory, people develop schemas that function as anticipatory mechanisms that help them interpret themselves and their social world. Moreover, people vary in the extent to which they adopt masculine and feminine schemas. Bem (1981) argued that people with sex-typed gender schemas rely on stereotypic dimensions of masculinity and femininity. Her findings reveal that they recognize stereotypic word pairings (e.g., bikini/nylon), and they more quickly label themselves with stereotypic terms.

Similarly, Maccoby and Jacklin (1974) suggested that the centrality of one's "masculine" or "feminine" gender role identity can moderate presumed sex differences. Maccoby and Jacklin argued, "If the studies summarized in previous chapters of this book had been based on selected subsamples of subjects, including only those women who consider it important to be feminine and those men for whom masculinity is central to their self-concept, the chances are that greater sex differences would have been reported and the findings would have been much more consistent than we have found them to be" (p. 360).

But if the answer is "no, the actor's sex-relevant beliefs are not stereotypic," then effects due to sex (matching the stereotype) cannot be readily predicted. If the answer is "yes, the actor's sex-relevant beliefs are stereotypic," we proceed.

3. *Are other contextual and/or individual moderators present?* Many contextual moderators exist and include a wide range of factors, such as the familiarity of the situation, the topic of conversation, and appropriateness rules. For example, Eagly and Johnson (1990) noted that "behavior may be less stereotypic when women and men who occupy the same managerial role are compared because these organizational leadership roles, which typically are paid jobs, usually provide fairly clear guidelines about the conduct of behavior" (p.

234). Moreover, the multitude of other situational factors that moderate sex-difference effects on power-related communication behaviors reflect a crossed effect (i.e., flipping the hypothesized effects due to sex; see also Chapter 4). For example, Instone, Major, and Bunker (1983) reported that men used a greater frequency of compliance-gaining strategies in an experiment involving stranger subordinates. However, Putnam and Wilson (1982) found that women used more controlling strategies when in familiar organizational surroundings versus unfamiliar organizational settings.

Individual moderators are plentiful. Directly relevant to our discussion is that one's sex role identity affects one's interaction behavior. Bem (1981) found that sex-typed individuals responded variously to attractive versus unattractive members of the opposite sex—more than did cross-sex-typed, androgynous, or undifferentiated people. Specifically, sex-typed individuals displayed more animation, interest, and enthusiasm toward attractive confederates. Bem concluded, "It appears, then, that the sex-typed individual may have a generalized readiness to code members of the opposite sex in terms of sexual attractiveness and that this readiness may be powerful enough to influence his or her social behavior in spontaneous social interaction" (p. 362).

4. *Does the relationship between the actor and the partner entail alternative expectations?* As indicated above, Fitzpatrick (1988a) has shown how different types of relationships promote alternative communication behaviors, suggesting that sex differences are moderated by these relational types. Fitzpatrick has demonstrated that "Separates" (who value autonomy and dislike expressing information or emotion) withdraw from conflict, whereas Independents (who balance autonomy with interdependence and negotiate their sex roles) readily engage each other in conflict, and Traditionals (who ascribe to conventional roles and prize interdependence) engage each other over important relational issues. Accordingly, we would expect to find nothing to support the sex stereotype hypothesis in a sample of Independent couples, whereas conventional sex differences should emerge more clearly for Traditional and Separate couples (e.g., the demand–withdrawal pattern, where the wife complains and the husband stonewalls; Christensen & Heavey, 1990).

In addition to this literature, it appears obvious that specific knowledge about the partner increases over time to allow more accurate explanation and prediction of the other's beliefs (Deaux & Lewis, 1984; Perlman & Fehr, 1987). An increased ability to predict a partner's response would give one greater confidence in responding strategically to one's partner, thus moderating sex differences. An increased ability to predict idiosyncratic behaviors of one's intimate partner also suggests that stereotypic responses occur mostly among strangers and acquaintances. Unfortunately, research on sex differences has largely relied on strangers, as Aries (1996) observed: "These data suggest that [sex] differences are more likely to be greatest in magnitude in initial interactions among strangers and may be mitigated when people get to know and interact with each other more extensively. Because the majority of research on [sex differences in] interaction has been carried out on strangers in brief encounters, we may tend to find more evidence for [sex] differences" than if partners in close relationships participated in the research (p. 37). Aries's comment implies that one should not generalize from strangers to intimates with regard to sex differences in interaction behavior. Nevertheless, if one believes that relational expectations do not alter people's general stereotypic responses, then one must continue the search.

5. *Does the partner's behavior promote a stereotypic response?* Deaux and Major (1987) noted that people follow each other's cues in interaction and that interdependence of responses can reinforce or revise stereotypic behavior. The influence of one person's behavior on the partner's is very strong and researchers are increasingly realizing the importance of studying behavior sequences. Burggraf and Sillars (1987) found that one's marriage partner's immediately preceding behavior strongly predicted one's own conflict behavior such that effects due to sex were nullifed by the partner's behavior. Likewise, Fisher (1983) examined whether sex or competition/cooperation orientations affected dyadic interaction behaviors. Fisher found that topic importance and competitive/cooperative orientations "swamped" interactional differences due to sex. It appears that the partner's behavior provides an immediate frame of reference for one's interaction behavior, overriding the more "foundational" influences on interaction behavior, including sex.

Some authors argue that stereotypes are widely held and prompt people to conform to expectations implied by the stereotype in a self-fulfilling manner (Geis, 1993). At a social level, interactions exist wherein stereotypic responses may prevail and reinforce gender stereotypes (Deaux & Major, 1987). But the extent to which the self-fulfilling nature of stereotypes extends into personal relationships remains unclear, though we acknowledge that it happens. Geis (1993) noted that education about stereotypes and currently shifting occupational roles of men and women can counterbalance the self-fulfilling nature of stereotypes. One should be able to locate where the enactment and perception of stereotypic behavior occur in interaction that might prompt a stereotypic response. Whereas the data appear to support a few *general* trends among acquaintances regarding stereotyping and self-fulfilling behavior, the literature does not reveal specific stereotypic communication behaviors in close involvements. We question the assumption that stereotypic responses typify interaction in close, personal relationships (see also Duck & Wright, 1993).

OVERVIEW OF THE PROJECT

The analysis we offer here is constrained in two ways. The first is that, although we examined research concerned with sex and gender differences in general, our specific population was people in close involvements. We were also constrained by the sheer amount of research on the topic of sex differences. Detailed reviews have been offered in many contexts and domains of behavior, including friendship (Fehr, 1996), marriage (Gottman, 1994), verbal interaction behaviors (Aries, 1996; Crawford, 1995), nonverbal interaction behaviors (Hall, 1984, in press), division of labor (Coltrane, 1996; Hochschild, 1989), and the like.

Moreover, sex differences in people in personal relationships have been approached from a variety of perspectives that we also cannot review here for lack of space, including psychological (e.g., Beall & Sternberg, 1993; Shaver & Hendrick, 1987), developmental (e.g., Maccoby & Jacklin, 1974), historical (Bem, 1993), social evolutionary (Kenrick & Trost, 1997), sociolinguistic (e.g., Tannen, 1993, 1994), cultural (Maltz & Borker, 1982), and critical (Thorne, Kramarae, & Henley, 1983), among others.[3] Our objective was to provide a fair representation of the literature that examines sex differences from a social scientific perspective. Realizing the above constraints, we attempted to synthesize what we believe to be the most relevant research bearing on the issue of sex differences in personal relationships. Although more recent research (vs. older studies) appears on the whole to have a more balanced orientation to the study of sex differences, we did not presume that recency equated with quality. In addition and unfortunately, in many instances, the "relevant" studies involved inferences made from strangers interacting or participants who report how they would *likely* behave in hypothetical scenarios involving their partners. Accordingly, although we sought studies that directly examine sex/gender differences in personal relationships, we also needed to rely on papers that only implicate what sex/gender differences would be in close involvements.

Finally, we want to stress that we assume that *communication* (i.e., the exchange of symbols between people) provides the primary mechanism whereby relationships develop and deteriorate (Hinde, 1976). As Duck (1994) observed, "Daily talk is not only a neutral medium or a simple expressive act but also an organizer of relational worlds in ways that sustain, maintain, and perpetuate them" (p. 142). Consistent with this assumption, we view gender differences in close relationships as a function of the process of two people communicating with each other over time. As Deaux and Major (1987) observed, "The enactment of gender primarily take place within the context of social interaction, either explicitly or implicitly" (p. 370). Metaphorically speaking, something about relating as a *process* diminishes many of the effects that people attribute to biological sex, much like the ocean eventually washes away structures on the beach.

We begin our review in Chapter 2 on the fundamental issue of whether or not men and women have different affective orientations. The primacy of emotional responses to personal relationships is made quite clear in research literature reviews (e.g., Andersen & Guerrero, in press; Gottman, 1994). Moreover, emotions need to be expressed as well as experienced (Andersen & Guerrero, in press). Presumably, people enjoy positive emotions in their personal relationships (Planalp, 1992). Of course, however, people experience a variety of emotions that may affect their interactions and relationships. We review five fundamental emotional responses and potential sex and gender differences to them: fear, anger, sadness, joy, and love.

Chapters 3 and 4 concern two dimensions of interpersonal interaction that are critical to personal relationships: *intimacy* and *control* (Burgoon & Hale, 1984; Leary, 1957). In terms of dimensions important to personal relationships *and* sex/gender differences in personal relationships, the literature strongly suggests that intimacy (Chapter 3) and control (Chapter 4) qualify as the most salient dimensions of relational life wherein sex/gender differences may exist. Increased interdependence found in personal relationships requires that the parties coordinate their plans and activities, which in turn requires one or both parties to provide structure and leadership in couple decision making (Braiker & Kelley, 1979). The reviews we offer are contextualized by other reviews on sex and gender differences in intimacy (e.g., Fehr, 1996) and power (e.g., Kalbfleisch & Cody, 1995).

Chapter 5 discusses the division of household labor. Hochschild (1989) observed, "The second shift becomes a forum for each person's ideas about gender and marriage and the emotional meanings behind them" (p. 188). According to Eagly's (1987) theory of social roles and gender, people learn how to assign gender roles within the context of the division of labor. And other scholars (e.g., Berk, 1985) have argued that the home provides the context wherein gender is created because that is where labor assignments are made and learned.[4] In other words, people's gender role identities become established early in the home and in relation to the performance of those household chores that are often sex stereotyped.

An alternative corpus of literature concerns a secondary sphere of activities relevant to gender construction: play and leisure activities (i.e., nonworking time). For instance, Maccoby (1988, 1990) has reviewed the literature concerning the sex-segregation hypothesis in showing that boys' play and girls' play represent different forms of behavior that lead to differentiated understandings of each other as groups. However, play appears to complement the primary sphere of activity, the division of labor; Firestone and Shelton (1988) referred to leisure time as "residual time, " or how one spends time not devoted to working, sleeping, and eating (p. 480). In addition, the content of play and leisure appear to be affected more by the division of labor than vice versa. This is illustrated in how young children role play alternative careers (e.g., boys play "doctors" and girls play "nurses"), and in the many toys that reinforce the existing division of labor (e.g., G.I. Joe figures for boys vs. girls playing with doll houses). We do not review the play or leisure time research in depth in any one chapter, although we discuss it as a secondary sphere of activities that define gender (Chapter 6).

Finally, in Chapter 6, we offer our emerging view of sex and gender differences: With regard to personal relationships and communication behavior, men and women are not from different planets. Rather men and women originate from the same planet and define their genders in terms of goal-directed activities. In a word, gender refers to a cluster of activities that reveal different prototypes of men and women. Our discussion does not rely on historical or critical views, though we find such reviews rich with insight (e.g., Bem, 1993; Coltrane, 1996). Rather, and consistent with the remainder of the book, we rely on social scientific theory and research to make our points.

CONCLUSION

Many social scientific researchers have examined sex and gender differences in interaction behavior for the past 50 years, though much of this research perpetuates stereotypic thinking of how men and women communicate in their personal relationships. Feminist reactions to sex differences have generally taken two routes, to deny difference or to celebrate women's differences. The meaning of difference has been problematic at best, restricting opportunities for both men and women and ignoring their experiences (Rhode, 1990).

Some people assume that differences between men and women reflect stable predispositions, leaving out potentially more important aspects of individuals and culture. In addition, as Deaux and Major (1990) stated, "Dualistic assumptions about gender may also preclude other relevant categories—race, class, age—from entering the analysis" (p. 89). We hope to locate places when difference should be questioned and when it should be celebrated. In our view, the quality of our close relationships depends on increased understanding of sex differences and similarities as well as the activities that reflect people's gender.

2

❖

Sex, Gender, and Emotion

We believe it is appropriate early on to examine the relationship of sex, gender, and emotion. Experiential and expressive aspects of emotion reside in individuals as social actors, and they are central to how people get along in their personal relationships. In addition, the experience and expression of emotion provide a useful background for understanding how sex differences and similarities emerge in personal relationships. In other words, emotions present a valuable frame of reference for later discussions of men's and women's behaviors regarding intimacy, control, work, and play. We begin this chapter by exploring definitional premises of emotion; briefly discussing methodological issues; reviewing the literature on men, women, and emotion; and concluding with a synthesis of the more relevant findings.

DEFINING AND CHARACTERIZING EMOTION

Emotion is a blanket term, covering multiple physiological experiences, feelings, and expressions. Akin to a quilt, emotions resemble numerous converging patches with varying representations and intensities. Some emotions are strong, pleasing, and reinforcing whereas others haunt, taunt, and erode our well-being. If we fail to manage emotional highs and lows, particularly in the context of our close personal relationships, this may very well contribute to our being "torn at the seams," to extend the metaphor. At the relational level, emotions must somehow be conveyed to the partner; such expression can take the form of individual responses and relational commentaries (Andersen & Guerrero, in press). Similarly, theoretical explanations of sex differences in emotional developmental processes connect emotions to their interpersonal expressions (Brody, 1985).

Although everyone knows that *emotion* exists, people experience difficulty defining the term (Fehr & Russell, 1984). For instance, Lee (1974) argued that one of the most difficult tasks facing two people is defining the emotion of love. Although many couples might never explicitly define "love," partners likely consider the meaning of the emotion nonetheless. Often, partners' definitions of love do not coincide; for example, whereas one person may define love as "passion and chemistry," the partner may define it as "friendship" (Lee, 1974). Overall, emotions reference something that people undoubtedly experience, yet individuals may or may not attempt to isolate emotions into a comprehensible form.

Regardless of lay understandings of emotion, investigating men's and women's experience and expression of emotion, particularly in personal relationships, merits pursuit. Some scholars argue that increased understandings of emotion can be applied to personal benefit. As stated by Planalp (1992), "One of the most important functions of emotions is to guide us toward happiness, most importantly through our close relationships" (p. 21). Still, *defining* emotion remains a challenge.

Emotions can be regarded as ubiquitous and constant, varying in degree of strength and valence (Metts & Bowers, 1994). Alternatively, emotions can be characterized as phenomena elicited from a base state due to interruptions in usual patterns of behavior (e.g., something occurs during a typical day that arouses anger) (Vangelisti, 1994). Yet, scholars cannot agree on a definition of *base state.* Some researchers regard emotions as internal states (i.e., properties inherent in the individual), whereas others view emotions as products of social relationships (i.e., constructed through interaction) (de Rivera & Grinkis, 1986), as an expression of individuals to society in general (Radley, 1988), or as social constructions (i.e., "society" constructs meanings associated with various emotions and appropriate affective and behavioral responses that result from experience of such emotions) (Kippax, Crawford, Benton, Gault, & Noesjirwan, 1988). Other researchers argue that emotions are difficult to distinguish from each other. Scherer and Tannenbaum (1986), for instance, found only the emotions of happiness and anger as "pure" states and other emotions, such as sadness and fear, blended with other emotions (see also Berkowitz, 1993).

Fundamental and Discrete Emotions

Whereas Scherer and Tannenbaum (1986) isolated "pure" states, Izard (1991) separated fundamental emotions from discrete emotions. Izard proposed five characteristics of fundamental emotions: (1) distinct and specific neural substrates, (2) a distinct and specific configuration of facial movements or facial expressions, (3) a distinct and specific feeling that achieves awareness, (4) evolutionary–biological processes, and (5) organizing and motivational properties that serve adaptive functions (p. 49). Izard argued that the emotions of interest, enjoyment, sadness, surprise, anger, disgust, contempt, and fear meet these five standards of fundamental emotions (p. 49). Other emotions that do not meet these criteria, such as love, represent discrete emotions.

Components of Emotions

Whereas some definitions treat emotions as an encompassing blanket term, other definitions stress various emotional aspects (e.g., the expressive vs. the experiential). One theory that conceptualizes emotions as holistic, independent, and/or interdependent components is *differential emotions theory* (Izard, 1991). Strongly influenced by Tompkins (1962, 1963), the theory defines *emotion* as "a complex process with neural, neuromuscular/expressive, and experiential aspects" (Izard, 1991, p. 42). Because this chapter reviews research examining emotion at the neural (e.g., heart rate, hormonal release), expressive (e.g., facial, glandular, gestural, and vocal aspects), and experiential (e.g., motivating experience and the associated meaning) levels, we find this encompassing definition of emotion to be appropriate. We are not suggesting that this is the only viable or preferred theory on emotion. We are suggesting, however, that differential emotions theory provides an inclusive explanation for various aspects of emotion that have been studied.[1] Although differential emotions theory assumes 10 fundamental emotions, much of the research on emotion has focused on 5 prototypic emotions (fear, anger, sadness, joy, and love) (e.g., Fehr & Russell, 1984; Shaver, Schwartz, Kirson, & O'Connor, 1987), and these 5 prototypic emotions are included in differential emotions theory's schemata (Izard, 1991). The *presence* of these emotions relative to men and women, however, depends on the method used to measure emotion.[2] The next section briefly explores the implications of using various methods to examine emotional aspects.

METHODOLOGICAL CONCERNS

Planalp (1992) posed the general question regarding the association of cognition and emotion: "Should we speak of cognition in opposition to emotion or in conjunction with it?" (p. 1). According to Izard (1991), emotions can be a direct product of neurochemical and affective processes independent of cognition. Thus, we must examine *how* emotions are measured. Second, we must consider the use of language in reporting research results.

Measuring Emotions with Self-Report Data

Researchers can examine emotions physically (e.g., heart monitor, hormonal monitoring), experientially (e.g., have participants self-report their feelings), or affectively (e.g., record observations indicative of individuals' emotional expression). Thus, the method used to examine emotions, then, would likely find emotional evidence *if* the method was conducive to the element(s) of emotion being examined (i.e., neurochemical, experiential, affectional). Specifically, the detection of emotion in research is not necessarily determined by the emotion's true existence; rather, it is typically indicated by the method or instrument utilized. Accordingly, the choice of emotional aspect (i.e., neurochemical, affectional, experiential) is an issue when considering an appropriate measure.

Measuring Emotions with Observational Data

Consider, too, the tenets of differential emotions theory (Izard, 1991) with individuals' use of self-monitoring behavior (e.g., Snyder, 1987) and face management techniques (e.g., Ekman & Friesen, 1978). The implications of these considerations suggest that the causal connection between *experience* and *expression* cannot be assumed. For example, recent research on affective orientation indicates that affectively oriented individuals are aware of their emotional states, value that information, and use that information to maneuver social interaction (Booth-Butterfield & Booth-Butterfield, 1995, p. 331). Similarly, Ekman, Friesen, and O'Sullivan (1988) also argue that emotional expression can be manipulated, feigned, or suppressed. Thus, the bridge between experience and expression can vary from strong to nonexistent, depending on level of affectual orientation and/or cognitive connection with the expressive and physical elements.

According to Brody and Hall (1993), "though there is obvious merit in separating the experience of an emotion from its expression, not all research permits clear distinction" (p. 448). In that vein, another problem with emotion research is that researchers' language often implies the unidimensionality among emotions (i.e., the terms "experience" and "expression" are used synonymously). Therefore, to assume conceptual symmetry among neurochemical, experiential, and expressive aspects or a causal connection among the concepts (i.e., experience causes expression; neurochemical existence and expression cause cognition) is both presumptuous and, sometimes, erroneous.

RESEARCH ON SEX, GENDER, AND EMOTION

This section reviews various research examining men and women and the prototypic emotions of fear, anger, sadness, joy, and love. To begin, we examine the emotion of "fear." As the following section will illustrate, men's and women's conceptualization and experience of fear can vary. These variations may hold serious implications regarding partners' inclinations about the relationship, their significant other, and themselves. In addition, these inclinations are likely manifested in the partners' interactions (or may be associated with the lack of interaction).

Men, Women, and Fear

Much of the research on men's and women's experience of fear indicates that women experience fear more frequently than men (e.g., Chambless, 1982; Stafford & Galle, 1984; Warr, 1984). However, men and women may have different conceptualizations of fear. For example, Lohr, Hamberger, and Bonge (1988) found that, when examining physical injury factors, men viewed physical injury as pertaining to damage to oneself or one's property. Women, on the other hand, had more of an emotional conceptualization of physical injury. Specifically, women viewed being *physically* injured as being "treated unfairly or being taken advantage of by others" (p. 179). Blier and Blier-Wilson (1989) found that women feel more confident than men expressing fear to both men and women.

Research has produced conflicting findings regarding the effects of sex (i.e., biological aspects) and gender (i.e., social constructions of gender roles) on experienced fear. From a sex role standpoint, some research suggests that men experience more physical manifestations of fear that are reflected in their health problems (Dillon, Wolf, & Katz, 1985). Others argue, however, that women experience more fear from a gender standpoint (Bankston, Thompson, Jenkins, & Forsyth, 1990). That is, one's identification with a feminine gender role associates with higher reported fear, whereas identification with the masculine gender role associates with lower reported fear.

Contrary to gender role stereotypes, Levenson, Ekman, and Friesen (1990) found autonomic differences among the negative emotions of anger, fear, disgust, and sadness as opposed to the positive emotions of happiness and surprise. However, they found no significant autonomic differences among emotions between men and women.

Nevertheless, much of the research available examines men and women from a gender role standpoint. For example, Dillon et al. (1985) examined how men and women experienced fear using Bem's (1974) four gender role categories (masculine, feminine, androgynous, and undifferentiated). Using self-report data, Dillon et al.

found that women scored higher than did men in fear. However, gender role contributed equally to the variability across scores. That is, men's and women's scores in the masculine, feminine, androgynous, and undifferentiated categories were equally affected by their sex roles.

Often, people confront situations that induce fear. This concept can be separated into *fear for ourselves* (personal fear) as well as *fear for others* (altruistic fear) (Warr, 1992). Much of past research has indicated that women experience more personal fear than men (e.g., Warr, 1984). Given traditional stereotypes of women being more nurturing and caretaking than men, Warr expected that women (vs. men) experience more altruistic fear for household members. However, Warr found that *men* experienced more altruistic fear for their household members (49%) than women did (41%). Interestingly, 33% of men experienced altruistic fear for their wives, whereas only 10% of the wives experienced altruistic fear for their husbands. In regard to children, however, women experienced more altruistic fear than did men (38% vs. 11%, respectively). Consistent with gender and sex role stereotypes, Warr concluded that these results support the notion that women are responsible for the welfare of children and view men as being able to care for themselves.

Whereas Warr (1992) argued that women may view men as stronger and, therefore, able to take care of themselves, Eagly and Steffen (1986) offer an alternative reason as to why women may not view themselves as strong or aggressive. In a meta-analysis, Eagly and Steffen (1986) found that women experienced anxiety and fear about possible *outcomes* of being forthright and aggressive. This explanation partially supports Warr's (1984) finding that women experience more fear for their personal safety than do men.

According to Nicholson (1993), however, there is fault in the popular operationalizations of fear as it is examined in sex difference research. Specifically, items in many of the measures reflect situations that women would likely find frightening whereas men would not (e.g., items that reflect threats to personal safety because women are typically not as physically strong). When examining research on "sex differences," then, one should consider whether the researchers examined sex differences or differences found due to social constructions or adaptation to stereotypes. The previously reviewed research seems only to find differences when stereotypical gender roles are at the heart of the research. Research examining true sex differences (e.g., Levenson et al., 1990) found no differences between men and women; rather, they only found differences in the emotions themselves.

Fear and Personal Relationships

Regarding the reviewed research on sex, gender, and fear in personal relationships, several interpretations can be drawn. From a sex role standpoint, fear has been shown to contribute to more health problems in men than women (e.g., Dillon et al., 1985). Warr (1992) found that husbands experience more fear for their wives' well-being than wives experience for that of their husbands. Perhaps then, the pressure associated with men's perceived efficacy at fulfilling the "strong and capable" masculine gender roles takes its toll.

Men involved in close relationships may feel the impact of this gender role expectation more than men uninvolved in personal relationships. Specifically, men in close relationships often experience more barriers to relational dissolution (Attridge, 1994). A man's fear of failing to uphold his role, then, holds implications for himself, his significant other, his relationship, and other structural aspects of personal relationships (e.g., financial obligations).

Research also suggests that men experience more difficulty expressing fear than women (Blier & Blier-Wilson, 1989). One may believe that inclusion in a close relationship provides men a safe haven for emotional expression due to the intimacy and comfort associated with many personal relationships. According to Gottman (1994), however, men in close relationships often withdraw and otherwise avoid discussing important relational issues due to the "flooding" they feel when confronted. Conversely, women typically express their feelings with more confrontational and hostile affect (Chapter 4). In the context of close relationships, then, it appears that both men and women experience fear and that identification with one's gender role relates to the expression of fear (Warr, 1992). Women, as a group, appear to have more latitude in expressing their feelings, including fear (e.g., Blier & Blier-Wilson, 1989; Gottman, 1994).

Men, Women, and Anger

In a recent review of sex differences in how people manage anger in their personal relationships, Cupach and Canary (1995) found many more similarities than differences. For instance, the causes for anger are largely the same—both men and women bristle at condescension and lack of fair treatment. Frost and Averill (1982) also concluded that "as far as the everyday experience of anger is concerned, men and women are far more similar than dissimilar" (p. 297).

In addition, men and women appear to use more similar, rather than dissimilar, kinds of communication messages (Cupach & Canary, 1995). Cupach and Canary did find one nonverbal message that was used and interpreted differentially by men and women, that being tears: Women are more likely than men to cry when angry, and women interpret their tears as indicators of anger; whereas men are more likely to interpret tears as a sign of weakness. Still, given that sex similarities appear to outweigh differences in the antecedents to and expression of anger, one cannot presume that biological differences clearly predict the emergence of anger in personal relationships.

It is possible that one's gender role identity (vs. sex) plays a more substantial role in people's anger. In this vein, Eisler, Skidmore, and Ward (1988) argued that men's identification with the masculine gender role would contribute to elevated anger and stress in comparison to women. Using the Masculine Gender Role Stress questionnaire (MGRS), Eisler et al. hypothesized that men would experience more stress than women when attempting to live up to expectations linked to being a "male" or when immersed in a situation that required feminine behaviors. Results indicated that men do experience much more masculine gender role-related stress than do women. Moreover, both men and women who identified with the masculine gender role experienced elevated anger, stress, and health problems. Interestingly, the MGRS had no correlation with masculinity as measured by the Personal Attributes Questionnaire (PAQ) (Spence, Helmreich, & Stapp, 1974).

In a similar vein, Janisse, Edguer, and Dyck (1986) examined Type A behavior, anger, and sex on self-control and heart rate. Results from the self-report and heart rate data revealed complex interaction effects regarding sex and the other independent variables. For example, Type A males (not Type A females) high in anger expressiveness self-reported much more anger, generated more acute anger imagery, and had less perceived self-control than did Type A low-anger expressives, Type B high-anger expressives, and Type B low-anger expressives. Janisse et al. concluded that need for self-control may be a central need for Type A individuals and this need is driven not only by situational factors, but by proneness to anger expression as well as sex. This finding mirrors Emmons and Diener's (1986) assertion that different personality types (i.e., temperament) affect varying levels of emotion.

Research that examines physiology in married relationships indicates some sex differences. For example, Gottman and Levenson (1992) examined prototypic emotions revealed in speaker affect between married couples and how such processes were associated with marital dissolution over a 4-year period. Couples were classified as either regulated or nonregulated. "Regulated" couples' interactions were typified by both husbands' and wives' communication (measured by speaking slopes) being significantly positive. In "non-regulated" couples, at least one partner's communication was not significantly positive. Results indicated that husbands in regulated marriages compared to wives were more neutral, showed more affection, were less angry, and whined less. Gottman and Levenson noted that women often take the responsibility to regulate the affective balance in marriage by initiating negative affect. This initiation of anger is not necessarily relationally negative because it can generate discussions of problematic issues. In nonregulated couples, however, women/wives tend to intensify their anger, which can be dysfunctional to marital satisfaction and stability.

Other research reveals an inconsistent image of the experience and expression of anger in personal relationships. For example, Friedman and Miller-Herringer (1991) found that men were more likely to experience and exhibit anger nonverbally than were women. However, Noller (1982) found that wives (vs. their husbands) rely more on nonverbal displays of anger, including scowling and use of angry paralanguage. If findings regarding nonverbal messages appear contradictory, then perhaps sex differences reside in the perceptions of anger.

One study found no differences in men's and women's abilities to determine emotion from verbal descriptions of several situations and interactions (Dore' & Kirouac, 1985). However, Rotter and Rotter's (1988) examination of facial expressions eliciting the negative emotions of anger, disgust, fear, and sadness revealed that women more than men tended to identify successfully most emotions expressed by both sexes. The only exception was that men were better able than women to recognize male anger. Rotter and Rotter concluded that, for men, men's anger may be easier to identify than women's because men tend to externalize anger to each other whereas women internalize it.

In examining people's attributions for anger, Egerton (1988) hypothesized that women, unlike men, tend to attribute their anger to an external locus of control. Testing Averill's (1982) rule model of anger, Egerton examined norms of aggression possessed by the two sexes. According to this perspective, those who have strong norms against aggression are more likely to attribute their personal anger to passion. Typically, women fall into this category and are more likely to attribute their anger to an uncontrollable, outside force (e.g., "something came over me and I couldn't help myself"). Men, conversely, would more typically attribute anger to an internal locus of control (e.g., "I decided to make a strong impression"). Egerton (1988) predicted that women (vs. men) regard anger as more costly to norms and to the overall situation, and as more upsetting. Results indicated that women viewed the episode as being more costly to the relationship and to life-scripts (e.g., anticipated way of living, fulfilling roles, etc.), and as more upsetting. Women, contrary to stereotype, did not view the behavior as more unacceptable than did men. Interestingly, women gained satisfaction from engaging in the episode, although they were not more satisfied overall than men. This finding suggests that women feel situational and periodic triumph for achieving their goal; yet, their enthusiasm may wane once the role violation is recognized.

Lohr et al. (1988) also examined situational versus personal dispositions toward anger arousal. Specifically, they compared propensity for anger and irrational beliefs between men and women utilizing the Novaco Anger Scale (Novaco, 1975). Lohr et al. found sex differences in regard to situational anger arousal. For example, men more likely viewed *inconsiderate others* as being inconsiderate or obnoxious strangers, whereas women tended to view *inconsiderate others* as more familiar. Interestingly, men showed responsiveness to physical or chaotic situations (e.g., a fight) whereas women were responsive with anger in uncontrollable situations (e.g., a snowstorm). This finding parallels Egerton's (1988) assertion that women adopt stronger norms against aggression and would more likely attribute anger to uncontrollable forces. Lohr et al. (1988) concluded that, for women, anger-inducing situations may be affected by relational quality whereas, for men, the inducement of anger may be affected by the physical consequences of the interaction (e.g., elevated heart rate). Possibly, then, "feminine sex [gender]-role socialization involves the acquisition of irrational beliefs that serve to suppress anger expression because it may be perceived as gender-inappropriate" (Lohr et al., 1988, p. 182).

Anger in Personal Relationships

The reviewed research suggests that both men and women are affected by anger physically, experientially, and expressively. Unlike expressions of fear, research remains equivocal to sex differences in anger in personal relationships. Akin to expressions of fear, however, men and women who identify with the masculine gender role tend to experience more negative physical manifestations (e.g., elevated heart rate, stress; Eisler et al., 1988; Siegman, 1994) as a result of anger.

Within personal relationships, research indicates that how men and women manage anger is critical to the quality and stability of marriage (e.g., Gottman, 1994; Gottman & Levenson, 1992). Nearly two decades of research on how men and women in marital relationships express their anger indicates that competitive orientations and use of negative conflict messages erodes relational quality and stability (Canary, Cupach, & Messman, 1995). We return to the issue of sex differences in conflict management in Chapter 4.

We should also indicate that the experience and expression of anger are not divorced from other emotions. Berkowitz (1993) showed that people often act in an angry manner when responding to sadness or pain; for instance, women who performed a physically challenging task eliciting mild pain recalled more disruptive conflict interactions with their boyfriends than those who were not exposed to pain. Berkowitz argued that "any given emotional state is best regarded as an associative network in which specific types of feelings, physiological reactions, motor responses, and thoughts and memories are all interconnected" (p. 9). Anger could also be linked to other negative experiences such as stress or an aversive environment (e.g., overpopulated and hot conditions).

In addition, the emergence of anger in personal relationships can entirely moderate sex differences. For example, people vary in their temporary response tendencies in the way they manage their experience of anger (Frijda, Kuipers, & ter Schure, 1989). Perhaps more critically, people often reciprocate negative affect, including anger, which can override any effects due to sex differences (Burggraf & Sillars, 1987; Zillman, 1990). Recent research on violence shows that seeing physical violence as a principally masculine response to anger reflects a myth even more than research on sex differences suggests it does, largely because the experience and expression of anger in personal relationships is an interactional process involving both partners (Spitzberg, 1997).

Men, Women, and Sadness

As noted above, the experience of sadness can blend with other emotions (Berkowitz, 1993; Scherer & Tannenbaum, 1986). Other emotions, such as feeling depressed or angry, can contribute to feelings of sadness. Moreover, many regard experiencing low self-esteem or depression as "feeling sad."

Zuckerman (1989) examined sex differences in experienced stress and how that factor influences self-esteem, depression, and anxiety. Zuckerman found that, although both men and women experienced levels of stress, women reported more stress over mental health and familial relationships. This finding is consistent with Lohr et al.'s (1988) finding that women experience more anger than men over distress in close relationships. Zuckerman also found that men and women differed in how they manage stress. Women were more likely to feel depressed over the situation and were also more likely than men to vent their anger and express how they felt, consistent with Gottman and Levenson (1992). Zuckerman also reported that expressing anger and feelings was associated with lower coping and self-sufficiency and that men reported that they were higher in coping and self-sufficiency than women. When experiencing stress, men increased activity rather than becoming depressed. Interestingly, men who increased activity rated themselves higher on leadership and public-speaking ability. Zuckerman notes that increased activity by men under stressful situations was "inversely correlated with depression and is the only response pattern that was more common among the men than the women" (p. 442).

Friedman and Miller-Herringer (1991) examined men's and women's emotional expressiveness and high and low self-monitoring skills in social and solitary settings. Women were more expressive nonverbally (including sadness) than men. As noted earlier, however, men were more nonverbally expressive of anger than women. Conway, Giannopoulos, and Stiefenhofer (1990) examined the association between gender role orientation and sadness. Specifically, they examined actions taken by men and women when sadness was experienced. Consistent with sex stereotypes, the feminine gender role was associated with dwelling on sadness whereas the masculine gender role was associated with distraction when sadness was experienced. Women experienced more dwelling on the sadness than men and less distraction. Similarly, Zuckerman (1989) found that men increased activity when confronted with stressful situations whereas women became depressed.

Toner and Gates (1985) examined men's and women's decoding of facial expressions, including sadness expression. Specifically, they examined the effect of men's and women's emotional tendencies on their ability to decode facial expressions. Results indicated that women with inhibited, nonassertive personalities were less successful than more socially oriented females at emotional recognition. For men, the relationship between emotional disposition and identifying emotions was specific to particular emotions. For example, men's dispositions were related only to identifying anger, fear, surprise, and disgust.

Sadness and Personal Relationships

As with the previously discussed emotions, the implications of this research on sadness in personal relationships likely rest on how the sadness is managed during interaction. Men's and women's management of sadness suggests that women more typically internalize and dwell upon sadness, and such continuous contemplation can contribute to depression and stress (e.g., Conway et al., 1990; Zuckerman, 1989). Men, on the other hand, are more likely to avoid confronting their sadness by diverting their attention to other activities and chores (e.g., Conway et al., 1990). Thus, although women may be more nonverbally expressive of sadness than men, both women and men can avoid verbal venting of sadness through internalization and attention diversion, respectively.

At this point, the interplay of these alternative sadness coping styles with personal relationship maintenance remains ambiguous. That is, it is possible that avoiding momentary bouts of sadness through diversions like watching television, reading (nonacademic) literature, and physical exercise can help relationships indirectly through the individual's recovery from sadness. It does, however, appear that ongoing, chronic sadness can not be ameliorated through diversions (Canary & Spitzberg, 1993).

Men, Women, and Joy

Joy may be the most frequently experienced pure, prototypic emotion (Scherer & Tannenbaum, 1986). Joy is a positive emotion, though it is different than sensory pleasure (Izard, 1991). As with other emotions, both men and women experience joy. Expressions of joy, often captured through facial expression (e.g., Ekman & Friesen, 1982), continue to be studied and are considered to be pan-cultural (e.g., Ekman & Friesen, 1986). From a physiological standpoint, however, joy has not been studied extensively (Izard, 1991). Nevertheless, some research (e.g., Ekman, Levenson, & Friesen, 1983) has found heart rate and bodily temperature changes to distinguish joy from other emotions.

In a comprehensive review of research examining sex differences in general happiness and well-being, W. Wood, Rhodes, and Whelan (1989) found that women (vs. men) tended to report more happiness and life satisfaction. Well-being and happiness were shown to be due to marital status. W. Wood et al. concluded that the gender differences regarding happiness were related to the idea that the feminine gender role calls for greater emotional responsiveness. Similarly, from a sex difference standpoint, Delp and Sackheim (1987) explored men's and women's emotional responsiveness and found that women's propensity to cry significantly decreased after a happiness manipulation (and increased following a sadness manipulation). Mood manipulation, however, did not significantly affect tearing or crying in males.

In a related study on moods, Wessman and Ricks (1966) examined feelings associated with joy. (But according to Izard, 1991, how they defined *mood* "seems rather similar to the concept of emotion trait in differential emotions theory" [p. 171].) Wessman and Ricks developed and administered their Personal Feelings Scales to both men and women to examine the highest levels of elation experienced by four personality types (i.e., happy, unhappy, variable, and stable). The authors found that happy men and women experienced elation as a sense of verve, whereas unhappy men and women experienced elation as relief. Variable mood men and women experienced elation as happiness and inner peace, whereas stable men and women experienced elation as a state of serenity. Wessman and Ricks also found that fear, anger, and guilt manifested themselves in unhappy men's relationships, whereas happy men were more confident and outgoing, and they successfully experienced close relationships.

Not all research, however, has found sex differences in the experience of happiness. For example, Fujita, Diener, and Sandvik (1991) examined sex differences in affect and found no differences related to the experience of happiness. Similarly, Fugl-Meyer, Branholm, and Fugl-Meyer (1991) examined the impact of sex and age on happiness within a Swedish population. Although women were more satisfied than men in regard to relations with one's partner, family life, and sex, overall happiness was not affected by age nor sex.

Joy and Personal Relationships

According to some research (e.g., W. Wood et al., 1989), women's happiness is modestly associated with relational status (i.e., marriage). Similarly, happy men (vs. unhappy men) experience closer and more satisfying relationships (Wessman & Ricks, 1966). Wessman and Ricks concluded that men's happiness begins developing through successful childhood experiences. According to Izard (1991), "biogenetic, socioeconomic, and cultural factors play a role in the development of the joy threshold" (p. 149). In addition, a lack of joy manifests itself in relationally destructive ways. Wessman and Ricks found that unhappy men's relationships were typified by fear, anger, and guilt. Moreover, unhappy men tended to be withdrawn and avoidant of interaction. Izard provided insight in the observation that we should consider biogenetic, socioeconomic, and cultural factors when examining the emotion of joy. (Indeed, such components could be considered when examining all aspects of emotion in respect to men and women.)

Men, Women, and Love

Experiences of love take on various forms (Hecht, Marston, & Larkey, 1994). Love can be defined as emotionally intense (e.g., passion, obsession) or emotionally stable and affiliative (e.g., closeness, attachment, companionship) (C. Hendrick & Hendrick, 1991). Research offers mixed findings regarding how men and women experience and express the emotion of love in close relationships. For example, Heiss (1991) examined men and women in love role definitions. He hypothesized that there would be sex differences in male and female intimate relationships such that women would be more other-oriented and men would dominate the relationship. Contrary to stereotype, results revealed that women were *not* more other-oriented. In fact, women assigned more other-orientation to men and less to themselves. Heiss concluded that this deviation from widely accepted gendered beliefs regarding the love roles of men and women may be due to the influx of the women's feminist ideologies within the sample of college students.

In surveying the feminist literature, Critelli, Myers, and Loos (1986) examined the relationship between gender role orientation and types of love experienced. Five different dimensions of love were examined (romantic dependency, communicative intimacy, physical arousal, respect for partner, and romantic compatibility). Results indicated that women subscribing to the feminine gender role scored high on romantic dependency, romantic compatibility, and respect. Men subscribing to the masculine gender role scored high on romantic dependency and romantic compatibility. Nontraditional females scored high on communicative intimacy but not respect (for partner), though they made favorable emotional statements. Nontraditional males scored high on communicative intimacy and respect. In accordance with the assumption that women are more emotionally expressive than males, women scored higher on overall communicative intimacy than did males. In brief, traditional males and females seem to adhere to romantic dependency and romantic compatibility dimensions of love, whereas nontraditional males and females appear to prefer communicative intimacy. Physical arousal, a biological dimension, was not associated with gender role orientation for males or females. From this, we can conclude that sex and gender do not necessarily go hand in hand.

In a similar manner, Bailey, Hendrick, and Hendrick (1987) examined how love styles and sexual attitudes are associated with masculinity and femininity. Their results supported popular beliefs regarding the association between gender roles and notions of love. Specifically, love as game playing (Ludus) positively related to masculinity and negatively related to femininity. Possessive and dependent love types (Manic) were positively related to femininity and negatively related to masculinity. Women were more pragmatic (Pragma) than men; that is, women had more practical, realistic notions of love. Finally, masculinity was unrelated to the attitudes of Eros (passionate), Storge (friendship/companionate), Agape (selfless), nor Pragma (practical). Femininity, on the other hand, was related to all six love types. Bailey et al. concluded that gender role orientation is a strong predictor of sexual attitudes and love. This notion is further explored in Chapter 3.

In a later study, C. Hendrick and Hendrick (1991) examined sex differences within the framework of five love dimensions (passion, closeness, attachment, manic love, and practicality) within a college sample. As expected, and similar to earlier research, women had a higher propensity for closeness and practicality in their love relationships than men. Unlike earlier research, however, women also subscribed to more passion (Eros) than males. Hendrick and Hendrick concluded that college females might hold higher passionate love orientations than do college males. One could interpret this in terms of educated women no longer necessarily needing to subscribe to the traditional, stereotypic notion of seeking "stability" in a mate. Given that many women can and do support themselves, they may seek passion and chemistry in a relationship rather than financial security and dependency (cf. Kenrick & Trost, 1997).

Considering sex and love, Foa et al. (1987) tested the assertion that men differentiate between love and sex more clearly than do women. Overall, U.S. participants differentiated love and sex more than Swedish participants. However, within U.S. and Swedish cultures, women were more likely than men to combine love and sex. Similarly, when examining sexual intercourse, romantic love, and emotional intimacy as justifications for extramarital affairs, Glass and Wright (1992) found that women (vs. men) are more accepting of love, as opposed to sexual desire, as a justification for an extramarital affair. The authors concluded that women seem to adopt the belief that love and sex are interrelated and that being in love justifies sexual involvement, whereas men had a higher tendency to separate sex and love (Chapter 3 examines this issue in more depth).

In a longitudinal investigation, S. S. Hendrick and Hendrick (1995) examined sexuality and love in personal relationships. Findings provided support for both sex differences and sex similarities within the context of intimate relationships. Specifically, women were less permissive and instrumental in their attitudes toward sex than were men. Women were also more friendship oriented toward love than were men, and men were more game playing in regard to love. Moreover, women (versus men) were more inclined to be in love, value love, and love intensely; men, on the other hand, reported higher frequencies of being in love and as having more sexual and relational partners. Given these differences, Hendrick and Hendrick nevertheless pointed out that correlational analyses provided support for exploring sex similarities. Specifically, when examining sexuality, only 11 of 60 pairs of correlations revealed that men and women significantly differed. Of those 11 significant correlations, only 5 pairs of correlations involved r's greater than .30. The authors concluded that "men's and women's attitudes toward sexuality and relevant relationship variables are very similar" (p. 61).

Love and Personal Relationships

S. S. Hendrick and Hendrick's (1995) findings support commonly held sex stereotypes of men and women regarding sex and love (i.e., that men are promiscuous and women are more monogamous). In addition, their findings echo earlier research suggesting that men typically assume the responsibility for advancing sexual intimacy (e.g., Perper, 1985), whereas women assume the role of relational "gatekeeper" in terms of sexual intimacy (Allgeier & Royster, 1991). Yet such differences must be interpreted within the context of the similarities that have been found. For example, Hendrick and Hendrick's (1995) findings also provide little support for a powerful sex difference argument; men and women were statistically similar on 49 of 60 (82%) of the correlates of love. The majority of their findings support men's and women's similarities with respect to love and sex, which they suggest examining further.

In addition, evidence suggests that men and women who do not subscribe to conventional, traditional gender roles hold similar attitudes toward love. Specifically, college education and more nontraditional attitudes seemingly contribute to less gender-typed attitudes toward love and sexuality (e.g., Critelli et al., 1986; Heiss, 1991). There may be a shift from traditional to nontraditional in the beliefs that men and women hold with regard to the emotion of love. Specifically, traditional men and women seem to dwell more on the *experience* of love (e.g., romantic dependency, romantic compatibility). Nontraditional men and women, however, focus more on *expressions of love* (e.g., communicating intimacy; Critelli et al., 1986). Conventional couples, then, may be less inclined to express feelings of closeness for their partner and discuss their intimate relationship than nontraditional couples.

CONCLUSION

This chapter reviewed some of the representative research concerned with emotional tendencies of men and women in general. Responses to fear (e.g., Blier & Blier-Wilson, 1989), anger (e.g., Lohr et al., 1988), sadness (e.g., Conway et al., 1990), joy (e.g., W. Wood et al., 1989), and love (e.g., S. S. Hendrick & Hendrick, 1995) were reviewed. Generalizing from these findings to sex differences in personal relationships constitutes a challenge. Nevertheless, and keeping in mind that much of this literature remains outside the realm of personal involvements, we offer several inferences. These conclusions largely comport with Brody's (1985) observations concerning the social development of emotions, especially that women (vs. men) tend to express their emotions more, though such differences are contextualized by sex similarities.

Fear

Research suggests that although men and women may experience fear differently, these differences are not necessarily due to biological sex differences. Rather, the differences are probably due to men's and women's varied conceptualizations and perceptions of fear. However, biological differences can indirectly affect perceptions. For example, men typically are physically larger and stronger than women (Nicholson, 1993), suggesting why women (vs. men) fear more for their physical safety (Warr, 1984). Interestingly, however, feminine gender role identification is positively linked to fear (i.e., identification with a feminine gender role results in greater experienced fear than does identification with a male gender role; Bankston et al., 1990). When men and women experience fear, research suggests, they have varied ways of coping. Specifically, men are more likely than women to suppress fear, and such suppression can reduce the likelihood of their expressing fear, which in turn can contribute to withdrawal from discussing their feelings.

Anger

Research on men's and women's experience and expression of anger indicates that men and women in personal relationships tend to become angry and express anger in a similar manner (Cupach & Canary, 1995), though some research suggests a general tendency for men (vs. women) to express anger (Friedman & Miller-Herringer, 1991; Janisse et al., 1986). However, examining how anger manifests itself in personal relationships would lead us to deemphasize these personal sex difference tendencies in favor of an interactional point of view on how anger is conveyed in personal relationships (Spitzberg, 1997). Men's and women's causes of anger, responses to anger, and expressions of anger (with the exception of tears as a statement of anger for women) appear more similar than different in personal relationships.

As with the research on gender roles and fear, inferences made about men's and women's anger expression in personal relationships are sometimes erroneously related to men's and women's adherence to conventional gender roles in less intimate situations; for example, it is "manly" to be angry, so men express anger more readily in social relationships involving strangers and acquaintances. Similarly, it is not "ladylike" for a woman to express anger or negative affect in public. Yet, women typically initiate and engage in conflict (Gottman, 1994) and feel triumph during anger expression (Egerton, 1988). Women's gender roles in social (impersonal) situations suggest passivity (e.g., Lohr et al., 1988). However, the research reviewed here and in Chapter 4 shows that men and women appear to express anger with equal frequency in *personal* relationships in a similar manner, though women appear to be more confrontational, negative, and indirect. This last statement not only contradicts a stereotypic view of women, it also contradicts anecdotal observations of how men and women in close personal relationships are said to respond to each other (Tannen, 1990).

Sadness

Women (vs. men) more typically experience and internalize sadness, which can lead to depression and stress. In facing inequity in their personal relationships, for example, women appear to be more likely than men to respond with internally focused sadness and depression, whereas men respond with externally focused anger (Sprecher, 1986). Men more often avoid confronting their sadness by diverting their attention to activities and chores (e.g., Conway et al., 1990). The research also suggests that conforming to gender roles to manage sadness, though not necessarily personally or relationally healthy, can be sufficient for men and women in the short term. However, long-term consequences of failing to discuss feelings of sadness may be more detrimental. Specifically, men's coping with sadness through diversion and women's coping with sadness through internalization are manifestations of avoidance that can contribute over time to problems in the relationship.

Joy

Links exist between emotion experience and expression, and well-being for men and women alike. For example, happy men (compared to unhappy men) experience closer and more satisfying relationships (Wessman & Ricks, 1966). Conversely, lack of joy serves as a contributor to other emotional experiences and expressions, such as fear or anger. Wessman and Ricks found that unhappy men's relationships were characterized by fear, anger, and guilt. Such experiences contributed to men's avoidance of interaction, which has been implicated as detrimental to the maintenance and satisfaction of close relationships. However, sex differences in terms of the expression of joy cannot be readily determined.

Love

The research on love indicates that individuals hold varying views of love and respond in various ways to their partners when in love (e.g., S. S. Hendrick & Hendrick, 1995). The research does reveal some sex differences, though these should be cast within a broader net of sex similarities. Men tend to hold a higher propensity for sexual promiscuity, and women more often subscribe to monogamy. As well, within dating relationships, men typically assume the responsibility for advancing sexual intimacy, whereas women assume the role of "gatekeeper" in terms of sexual intimacy (Allgeier & Royster, 1991).

Not all of the research findings reviewed on men and women and love, however, support traditional gender role stereotypes; other personality and educational factors contribute to less sex-typed attitudes. Specifically, less traditional men and women are more likely to *communicate* intimacy and love (Critelli et al., 1986), whereas more traditional men and women are more likely to focus on the *experience* of it. Moreover, it appears that men and women do *not* differ in terms of what they consider to be prototypic manifestations of love (Fehr, 1993).

The research on men, women, and emotion suggests that, although sex similarities far outweigh differences in the experience of emotions, women appear to have a wider latitude of emotional expression than do men. Women more than men tend to discuss directly issues concerned with their fear, anger, and lack of joy; men more frequently rely on indirect means for expressing their emotions—such as avoidance during anger episodes or distraction in times of sadness. Less conventionally defined partners appear to have a wider latitude of emotional expression, probably due to not feeling constrained by traditional gender role expectations. Accordingly, the general emotional context presented here leads us to conclude that sex differences do exist in emotional expression, but these differences are not monolithic and must be tempered by an understanding of how interpersonal needs are communicated in personal relationships. In the next two chapters, we explore how men and women more precisely convey intimacy and control.

3

❖

Communicating Intimacy

As mentioned in Chapter 1, scholars largely agree on at least two fundamental dimensions of relational life—intimacy and control (Burgoon & Hale, 1984; Leary, 1955; Schutz, 1967). That is, some consensus exists that personal relationships can be profitably characterized in the degrees to which couples convey feelings of intimacy (or corresponding feelings, e.g., affiliation, affection, love) and deal with issues of control (or similar dynamics, e.g., power, influence, dominance). Of course, other relationship properties are important (e.g., commitment), but most researchers in the field of personal relationships appear to focus primarily on the dimensions of intimacy and control. A good portion of the theory and research on sex and gender differences in general has examined parties in personal relationships as opposed to other types of relationships. This chapter explores such differences (and similarities) in communicating intimacy, and the following chapter, in communicating control.

As with various emotions (e.g., love; Lee, 1974), *intimacy* remains difficult to conceptualize (Perlman & Fehr, 1987). Although scholars routinely view intimacy as a fundamental feature of close relationships, what is considered "intimate" varies. For instance, intimacy can reference understanding one's partner, interdependence, emotional closeness, or physical closeness. In addition, many studies presume alternative levels of intimacy among relationship type (e.g., friendship and platonic intimacy vs. romantic relationships and sexual intimacy), so pinpointing the *type* of intimacy variously experienced and communicated verbally and nonverbally in personal relationships presents a challenging exercise.

In this chapter we treat intimacy as an umbrella term for affiliative responses to the partner. According to Borisoff (1993), the nature of intimacy varies by relationship type, such as friendship, courtship, and marriage. Accordingly, this chapter focuses on intimacy in men's and women's same- and opposite-sex friendships and heterosexual dating relationships. More precisely, the following areas are explored: (1) representative conceptualizations of intimacy, (2) men's and women's same- and opposite-sex friendships, (3) heterosexual romantic relationships, and (4) sexuality.

DEFINING INTIMACY

Various definitions of intimacy exist (e.g., Acitelli & Duck, 1987; Hatfield, 1983, 1984; Perlman & Fehr, 1987; Prager, 1995). Intimacy can reference both an accomplished property or *product* of a personal relationship as well as a process. Perhaps assuming the first view of intimacy-as-product, scholars have examined behaviors and perceptions linked to different types of relationships that ostensibly vary in their levels of intimacy (e.g., Stafford & Canary, 1991). In the view of intimacy-as-process, scholars conceive of relationships as ongoing, "unfinished business" (Duck, 1990). According to Hatfield (1983), "Intimacy is not a static state, but a *process*. Intimacy may be defined as a process by which a couple—in the expression of thought, emotion, and behavior—attempts to move toward more complete communication on all levels" (p. 125, emphasis in original). We believe that intimacy as a construct for theory and research represents both a product of people's interaction (what partners have) and a process (what partners do).

Factors Associated with Intimacy

What factors relate to two people in intimate relationships engaging in "complete communication on all levels" (Hatfield, 1983)? Both men and women both utilize communication to achieve and express intimacy (Altman & Taylor, 1973), and self-disclosure serves as an exemplar of intimacy development (Perlman & Fehr, 1987; Prager, 1989). But self-disclosure is not isomorphic with intimate messages. Dindia (1994) showed in her review of relational escalation, maintenance, and deescalation strategies that people use self-disclosure to *decrease* as well as to increase intimacy. In addition, it is important to note that emphasizing disclosure predetermines the question of which sex engages in more "intimate" forms of communication, to the extent that emphasizing disclosure as an intimate activity is probably biased toward a feminine understanding of intimacy (J. J. Wood, 1993). Thus, although scholars often view self-disclosure as integral to intimacy development, numerous other factors and behaviors can affect the results regarding what people consider intimate.

Individuals usually recognize the cumulative experience of intimacy. Dissecting the experience, however, often proves to be more difficult. Specifically, one must question the defining feature of intimacy achievement: Is intimacy a function of psychological closeness (e.g., Miller & Lefcourt, 1982), of trust (Wong, 1981), of sexuality (e.g., Davis, 1973), of self-disclosure (e.g., Altman & Taylor, 1973; Perlman & Fehr, 1987), of commitment (e.g., Rusbult & Buunk, 1993)? Conversely, the *fear* of intimacy is said to reflect multiple dimensions, for instance, in the communication of information, evaluation of that information, and degree of vulnerability toward the partner (e.g., Sherman & Thelen, 1996).

In addition to establishing a primary defining feature of intimacy, one must consider the factors that cannot be "achieved" or manipulated by individuals. For example, it would appear that most people believe that time since onset of the relationship is positively linked to achieving intimacy, and accordingly a measurement of time serves as an indirect measure of intimacy. One might question the assumption that involvement in a long-standing relationship enables an individual to stake a greater intimacy claim than someone involved in a brief relationship or a one-night stand (presuming that intimacy varies by relationship type; Borisoff, 1993).

Another factor to be considered in reference to intimacy definition and experience is the *social construction* of intimacy and the impact of culture on intimacy in close relationships (Acitelli &

Duck, 1987; Ting-Toomey, 1991). Above and beyond the construction that may differ within, between, and among individuals, intimacy is also defined by culture. For example, Ting-Toomey (1991) found that individualism–collectivism, uncertainty avoidance, and masculinity–femininity affected expressions of love commitment, disclosure maintenance, ambivalence, and conflict among male and female students from the United States, France, and Japan. Specifically, individualism–collectivism affected love commitment and disclosure maintenance, uncertainty avoidance impacted conflict, and masculinity–femininity revealed sex differences in intimacy expressions within each of the three cultures.

Research into various cultures' ways of being also suggests that there is a paradox in the social construction of intimacy (Dion & Dion, 1993): individualistic cultures (e.g., the United States) often construct intimacy as romantic love and personal fulfillment; yet individualism seems to lessen the likelihood of realizing these relational aspects. Similarly, although collectivistic cultures value intimacy, their focus on family and other network relationships may inhibit the achievement of intimacy (Dion & Dion, 1993). Such incongruities are likely to affect how intimacy is achieved *within* a culture, and they are likely to affect how intimacy is achieved in close, *intercultural* relationships.

Measuring Intimacy

Given the amorphousness of the term "intimacy," it is not surprising that individuals characterize intimacy differently. Intimacy measures in the research reflect various ways in which to conceptualize and operationalize intimacy (e.g., Berscheid, Snyder, & Omoto, 1989; Miller & Lefcourt, 1982; Schaefer & Olson, 1981). Intimacy can be assessed from a number of dimensions, for instance, emotional, cognitive, and/or behavioral standpoints (Hatfield, 1983). Numerous measures of intimacy are available. Accordingly, we review a few of these in order to illustrate some of the various conceptualizations considered when measuring intimacy.[1]

Based on the notion of behavioral interdependence (e.g., Braiker & Kelley, 1979), intimacy would appear to require partners to have routine access to each other. Geographical proximity may be largely assumed such that partners can engage in activities together at will, with said activities largely operationalizing intimacy. Many items, for example, in Berscheid et al.'s (1989) Relationship Closeness Inventory appear to presume proximity and accomplishment of joint activities. However, there is research that indicates that geographically separated couples are capable of feeling *more* intimate and satisfied than those who enjoy geographical proximity (e.g., Stafford & Reske, 1990).

Psychological intimacy would appear to require an alternative approach to measures designed to assess behavioral interdependence. Miller and Lefcourt's (1982) Miller Social Intimacy Scale focuses on psychological closeness, that is, how close partners feel toward one another, which generally reflects cognitive and emotional factors. Along these lines, one might also measure psychological intimacy directly by assessing the extent to which an individual knows his/her partner *and* likes what he/she knows (Canary & Cupach, 1988). Accordingly, intimacy would appear to exclude relationships without much sharing of content, as well as negative and even neutral assessments that might accompany hostility or ambivalence about a partner who is well known to the self.

Specifying alternative experiences of intimacy, Schaefer and Olson's (1981) Personal Assessment of Intimacy in Relationships (PAIR Inventory) conceptualizes five facets of intimacy:

- *Emotional intimacy* reflects feeling close and being able to communicate openly and feel supported and understood.
- *Social intimacy* reflects having friends in common and social networks.
- *Sexual intimacy* involves physical closeness.
- *Intellectual intimacy* indicates being able to talk about various issues (e.g., work, life, current events).
- *Recreational intimacy* refers to partners' sharing in leisurely activities (e.g., sports or hobbies).

Considering the above, then, various conceptual and operational banners appear to be utilized to examine intimacy. Additionally, men's and women's "ways" of experiencing intimacy may alternatively be represented in the literature. To elaborate on this last point, the following section discusses two behaviors that scholars commonly identify as behavioral manifestations of intimacy: self-disclosure and touching.

TWO MANIFESTATIONS OF INTIMACY

Self-Disclosure

Theoretically, self-disclosure is a powerful tool for developing intimacy in personal relationships (Altman & Taylor, 1973). Although research supports women's use of self-disclosure (e.g., F. L. Johnson, 1996; F. L. Johnson & Aries, 1983b), there is less available evidence on men's use of self-disclosure. Recently, however, some researchers have argued that men utilize self-disclosure and expressiveness more than has been previously recognized (e.g., Inman, 1996). And we should point out that other researchers have questioned the importance of self-disclosure to the maintenance of relational intimacy, given that self-disclosure does not occur very often in people's daily, routine interactions (Duck, Rutt, Hurst, & Strejc, 1991).

Despite the above caveats, research has shown that self-disclosure predicts relational satisfaction for men and women in their same-sex friendships. D. C. Jones's (1991) research addressed the relation of intimacy (i.e., self-disclosure, trust, and affective tone) to friendship satisfaction. Relying on survey data, Jones expected that self-disclosure would be equally important to men and women in terms of their relational satisfaction. College women reported higher levels of self-disclosure, satisfaction, and less friendship negativity with same-sex friendships than did men. Reisman (1990) also found no support for the contention that men feel just as close to their same-sex friends as women. Indeed, in a meta-analysis of eight studies examining how meaningful (vs. superficial) college friendships are, Reis (in press) reports large effect sizes that show college women (vs. college men) as enjoying more intimate relationships.

Researchers should be cautious when interpreting results displaying landslides of difference in the depth of self-disclosure between men and women. "Research that emphasizes only distinctions in the magnitude of sex differences does not give sufficient attention to the qualities that promote satisfaction regardless of sex" (D. C. Jones, 1991, p. 181). A pertinent finding in terms of sex differences (and similarities) shows that for both men and women higher levels of reported self-disclosure and friendship enjoyment both contribute to friendship satisfaction (Jones, 1991). Men and women may use different standards for measuring the intimacy of their friendships (Caldwell & Peplau,

1982; J. J. Wood, 1993). In addition, Reisman (1990) observed that adolescent boys and girls expect to self-disclose in greater amounts to opposite-sex friends as they approach adulthood. The participants in his study also felt that the marriage relationship should be the most intimate. Self-disclosure can be viewed as a significant factor contributing to the satisfaction in same-sex friendships; sex matters little (cf., Sherman & Thelen, 1996). It remains that "having fun with friends and revealing personal information and feelings to friends heightens the sense of satisfaction with the friendship" (Reisman, 1990, p. 180).

When examining the domain of self-disclosure, more variables than the binary sex difference between men and women must be considered. "The original prediction that traditional male-role expectations inhibit men's disclosure is too simple because it does not take into account the many situational factors that affect disclosure" (Hill & Stull, 1987, p. 94). These authors examined the topics of disclosure, sex of target, and relationship to target, and they urged researchers to contemplate gender role attitudes, identity, and norms. Caldwell and Peplau (1982) reported, for instance, that women slightly preferred talking to doing activities in their same-sex friendships, whereas men preferred activities to talking (cf. Wright, in press).

Sharing emotions tends to characterize a lower percentage of men's than women's best same-sex friendships. Sollie and Fischer (1985) reported that women in their study disclosed most to their partners, followed by female and then male friends. The authors found that 38% of the variance was accounted for by target of disclosure. Support exists for the moderating effect of the topic of disclosure. Men prefer "masculine" content (e.g., adventure and aggression) when talking with male friends and are less likely to choose "feminine" content (e.g., personal concerns and vulnerabilities; Derlega, Durham, Gockel, & Sholis, 1981). However, this preference wanes when men talk with their women friends; in other words, men decrease their use of masculine content when disclosing to women friends (Derlega et al., 1981). As we report in the following chapter as well, men tend to accommodate more than women to their opposite-sex partner (i.e., men behave less stereotypically masculine).

Marital status, more than sex, appears to affect the extent of disclosure to same-sex friends. Tschann (1988) interviewed men and women concerning their disclosure to same-sex friends. She found that single (vs. married) people disclosed more about intimate topics. Women were relatively unaffected by marital status—they disclosed more intimate information to same-sex friends whether they are married or unmarried, whereas men who were married disclosed less about intimate topics and problems to their closest friends. Unmarried men and women, and married women appear to have the same patterns of self-disclosure to same-sex friends (Tschann, 1988). However, married men tend to disclose higher levels of intimate information to their wives, balancing low levels to close friends.

Friendships in which the parties assume feminine roles and in which males assume more androgynous roles are closer (e.g., G. P. Jones & Dembo, 1989), whereas men assuming masculine roles experience less intimate same-sex friendships (e.g., Aukett, Ritchien, & Mill, 1988; Jones & Dembo, 1989). Although women may prefer same-sex friendships over their opposite-sex friendships to fulfill intimacy needs, it is uncertain that this trend would hold in romantic relationships.

In relationships in which both partners have careers, the partners tend to be more similar in their communication. In fact, dual-career husbands reported disclosing more than their wives, contrary to differences hypothesized by researchers (Rosenfeld & Welsh, 1985). The study conducted by Rosenfeld and Welsh using data from questionnaires completed by both spouses in 30 dual- and single-career marriages assessed the difference in breadth, depth, and amount of self-disclosure. The reports of single-career couples indicate that wives disclose about more topics (breadth and amount) and express more intimate thoughts than their husbands. As well, dual-career husbands tend to report more depth of disclosure than do single-career husbands. As more people enter dual-career marriages, we may see more similarity in communicative acts such as self-disclosure. Stressful lifestyles and less conformity to traditional sex roles are major factors in more flexible and nontraditional sex communication roles.

Reasons for *not* disclosing generally can be affected by sex differences, though similarities between the sexes should be noted as well. According to Rosenfeld (1979), *both* men's and women's primary motivation for avoiding self-disclosure is fear of presenting an unwanted image of oneself. Secondary reasons for not disclosing revealed a few sex differences. Men's secondary reason for not disclosing concerned perceptions of losing control. Men's adherence to masculine gender roles, then, may hinder them from verbally expressing themselves due to perceived consequences of "not being strong." Women's secondary reasons for avoiding self-disclosure are to avoid personal and relational hurt (Rosenfeld, 1979). Burke, Weir, and Harrison (1976) also reported sex differences in reasons for withholding disclosures, though their study focused on marital relationships. Burke et al. found that wives more than husbands did not disclose in order to protect the spouse from worry (48% vs. 18%). More wives than husbands also reported that their spouses were relatively unresponsive to their personal problems (22% vs. 15%). Reflecting a traditional division-of-labor issue, husbands (vs. wives) reported that they withheld disclosure in order to separate work from home (25% vs. 0%) and because the spouse lacked the knowledge about the issue (20% vs. 0%). The Burke et al. findings, however, appear to reflect more on gender roles of the mid-1970s, when fewer women occupied work roles.

Finally, the effect of sex on self-disclosure cannot be discussed without the consideration of effect size and moderator variables. According to Dindia and Allen (1992), "The direction and magnitude of sex differences in self-disclosure varies systematically depending on these variables" (p. 113). The authors' meta-analysis of over 205 studies on sex differences in self-disclosure revealed that there are differences between men's and women's disclosure. However, these effects are moderated by the sex of the target, the respondent's relationship to the target (stranger vs. relationship), and the measure of self-disclosure (self-report vs. observation). Women disclosed, more than men did, to women, whereas men disclosed, more than women did, to men. However, in relationships, women disclosed more than men did. Dindia and Allen concluded that sex effects on self-disclosure are small (pp. 117–118).

An exclusive focus on differences between men's and women's self-disclosure in personal relationships is unwarranted. Rather, we need to direct our energy into understanding how circumstances (e.g., topic) and relationship type (e.g., egalitarian vs. traditional; dual- vs. single-career couples) interact with sex differences to affect self-disclosure.

Touching

Both men and women communicate intimacy through touch. One of the best-known examinations of same- and opposite-sex touch was Jourard's (1966) study, wherein he examined college students' use of touch among same- and opposite-sex friends and parents. He found that more parts of the body were touched in opposite-sex friendships than in same-sex friendships or in parent–child relationships. A replication of Jourard's (1966) study yielded results indicating even greater touch between opposite-sex friends (Rosenfeld, Kartus, & Ray, 1976).

In considering the use of touch in personal relationships, one should assess both private and public contexts. Clearly, increases in touch behavior between intimate partners occur within private settings, though partners' behavior in public also indicates intimacy. As one might anticipate, much of the research on public touch is based on observational methods (e.g., Guerrero & Andersen, 1991; Heslin & Boss, 1980), whereas the research on touch in private is based on self-report measures (e.g., Emmers & Dindia, 1995; K. Johnson & Edwards, 1991).

Research findings support both linear and curvilinear associations between relational intimacy and touch. For example, K. Johnson and Edwards (1991) examined commitment and various types of touch linked to increased intimacy: (1) hand holding, (2) kissing, (3) embracing, (4) upper-body petting, (5) lower-body petting, (6) heavy petting, and (7) intercourse. They found a linear association between relational commitment and touch. Conversely, when examining couples' touch in public, Guerrero and Andersen (1991) found a curvilinear association between relational stage and touch. Similarly, Emmers and Dindia (1995) found an asymptotic association between relational stage and touch when examining couples' touch in private.

Reinforcing the claim that women's verbal expressivity is more prevalent and normative than men's (e.g., F. L. Johnson, 1996), research also indicates that women's use of touch is more socially accepted than men's (S. E. Jones, 1986). When considering men's and women's use of touch in social settings or less advanced relationships, controversy exists regarding the intentions of and the messages conveyed by the behavior.

One existing argument is that men initiate more touch in opposite-sex relationships in order to express dominance and power (Henley, 1977). A rival hypothesis is that women initiate more touch due to their nurturing, expressive dispositions (S. E. Jones, 1986). Combining these two hypothesis would lead to the prediction of different expectations—both, however, are based on the presumption of sex differences. Another line of reasoning asserts that men's and women's touch patterns vary according to how advanced the relationship is. Some research indicates that women are more reserved haptically in early relational stages but become increasingly comfortable with touching as the relationship advances (e.g., Heslin & Alper, 1983; Heslin, Nguyen, & Nguyen, 1983). Other research, however, finds that men touch more in initial relational stages, but become increasingly reserved as relationships advance (Heslin & Alper, 1983). Emmers and Dindia (1995) found that both men and women reported touching their romantic partners similarly in frequency, but that women (vs. men) reported being touched more by their partners.

Whether or not one's sex constitutes a main effect apart from the relational context appears unclear. Within the context of close relationships, some research supports the popular notion that women communicate intimacy more than men do (e.g., Dosser, Balswick, & Halverson, 1986; Reis, Senchak, & Solomon, 1985). However, Hall and Veccia (1990) found no main effect sex differences in their meta-analysis on touch. According to Prager (1995), "There is evidence, then, that [sex] affects how much and what type of nonverbal intimate behavior will occur between interaction partners. At the immediate level, however, [sex] offers little in the way of explanatory value" (p. 187).

Explanations for sex differences and similarities in touching behavior often emerge from authors' acknowledgment of conventional sex roles in operation. For example, although Emmers and Dindia (1995) found some sex differences in perceptions of received touch, they noted that such differences were based on retrospective reports, which likely entail perceptual biases. Conventionally speaking, women are thought to be more affiliative and oriented to expression than are men (e.g., Exline, 1963; Street & Murphy, 1987). Accordingly, Emmers and Dindia argued that the "sex differences" they found in touching were possibly more perceptual than actual. That is, men in their study may have underreported being touched as much by their female partners because they were not as cognizant of receiving touch as were women.

In addition, adherence to gender roles may explain differences in men's and women's touch behavior (Eagly, 1987). Specifically, according to gender role theory, women are expected to fulfill structurally imbedded roles that require a communal and nurturing orientation. Accordingly, women would communicate more intimacy through touch, for instance, in opposite-sex relationships (Dosser et al., 1986; S. E. Jones, 1986; Reis et al., 1985). Men, on the other hand, are expected to fulfill roles that require an instrumental orientation, which might lead them to use touching as a method to influence or to control others (see also Henley, 1977).

FRIENDSHIPS

Problematically, various stereotypes exist regarding the closeness of men's and women's same- and opposite-sex friendships. For example, given the stereotype of men's preference for and comfort with minimized emotionality and expressiveness in relationships, one would expect men to favor same-sex friendships over opposite-sex friendships. Specifically, men "should" be more comfortable with relationships that perpetuate their "preference" for high instrumentality and low expressivity (i.e., relationships with other men). After all, stereotypically speaking, women's propensity for expressivity, self-disclosure, and emotionality should only make men uncomfortable. Similarly, one would expect women to favor opposite-sex friendships over same-sex friendships. The stereotype holds that women are competitive and jealous of other women (e.g., F. L. Johnson, 1996; La Gaipa, 1979). Thus, women may feel more useful and wanted, sharing their supportive and nurturing side, with opposite-sex friends who "need" an expressive female to bring them out of their shell. Contradicting this stereotype, however, is the notion that women enjoy (and prefer) self-disclosing with their same-sex friends.

Although such conceptions are doubtlessly stereotypical, such notions and images have been perpetuated for years. Interestingly, the research on men's and women's same- and opposite-sex friendships suggests something to the contrary of stereotypes. Although both men and women find happiness in friendship, research suggests that what makes men and women happy in their friendships can differ (Helgeson, Shaver, & Dyer, 1987).

Same-Sex Friendships

According to F. L. Johnson (1996), examination of women's same-sex friendships has suffered due to prevailing stereotypes (e.g., women are competitive, jealous, and catty). This is unfortunate, given that much of the existing research suggests that women tend to feel slightly more satisfied and comfortable with their female friends than men do with their male friends (e.g., Buhrke & Fuqua, 1987). Men, however, also experience close same-sex friendships. For instance, Booth and Hess (1974) reported that approximately 65% of men and 75% of women listed people of the same sex as their closest friend. Nevertheless, research suggests marked differences between men's and women's friendships. More specifically, although men's and women's friendships generally do not differ in terms of the number of friends, time spent with friends, or how much men and women value their friends, men's and women's friendships appear to differ in the experience and expression of intimacy (Aukett et al., 1988; Caldwell & Peplau, 1982).

Compared to men, women report more close friends and typically indicate that their close friends are of the same sex (D. C. Jones, Bloys, & Wood, 1990). Women's (vs. men's) same-sex friendships tend to be embedded in "talk" as a focal activity for conducting relationships (F. L. Johnson & Aries, 1983b), that is, women are said to achieve and to maintain intimacy in their close same-sex friendships through mutual sharing and disclosures (Caldwell & Peplau, 1982; Rawlins, 1992). From childhood through adulthood, females more typically engage in connectedness, interdependence, and intimacy in their same-sex friendships (e.g., Aukett et al., 1988; F. L. Johnson, 1996; F. L. Johnson & Aries, 1983a, 1983b; Rawlins, 1992, 1993).

Same-sex male friendships, however, appear to entail alternative actitivites relative to same-sex female friendships. Some of the prevailing research holds that, although men share satisfying same-sex friendships, men's friendships are often instrumental, based in physical activities (e.g., golfing) other than talk (e.g., Aries & Johnson, 1983; Aukett et al., 1988; Rawlins, 1992, 1993; Rose, 1985). One reason offered in the research for more physical and apparently competitive male activities concerns childhood play: Men engage more in team sports, for example (see also Chapter 6). A second reason provided for less intimacy in men's same-sex friendships is homophobia (Inman, 1996; Lewis, 1978). Problematic to some men, "intimacy" has long been defined by female standards as communal talk (J. J. Wood, 1993).

Inman (1996) argued that whereas much of the prevailing literature supports the notion that men's same-sex friendships are more instrumental and less expressive (e.g., Swain, 1989), recent research sheds new light on men's same-sex friendships (e.g., Duck, 1991; Duck & Wright, 1993). In particular, Inman observed that men's same-sex friendships are predominantly based on "continuity, perceived support and dependability, shared understandings, and perceived compatibility" (p. 100). These themes suggest that men's same-sex friendships are based more on perceptions and assumptions about the friendship than actual discussion and talk about the relationship. In addition, Inman found that men's same-sex friendships share nuances once thought to be more exclusive to women's same-sex friendships. Specifically, men's same-sex friendships also share "self-revelation and self-discovery, having fun together, intermingled lives, and assumed significance" (p. 100). Wright (in press) presented a similar analysis in noting that talk and shared activities both promote communality, as he illustrates with the example of two men playing chess on a routine basis and taking a weekend fishing trip. These activities suggest more connectedness and interdependence—themes typically deemed more specific to female same-sex friendships. Such findings suggest the emergence of a more expressive male than much of the prevailing literature portrays.

Other research nevertheless acknowledges the positive impact of self-disclosure and expressivity on intimacy achievement in men's and women's friendships (Camarena, Sarigiani, & Petersen, 1990). Similar to Inman's (1996) findings, G. P. Jones and Dembo (1989) found that a male's androgynous, expressive demeanor benefits intimacy development in childhood and adolescent friendships; individuals holding feminine gender identities experienced higher levels of friendship intimacy than those assuming masculine gender roles. Androgynous males experienced higher levels of intimacy in their friendships than males in masculine roles. Overall, females and androgynous males, compared to those holding masculine roles, form a cohesive, high-intimacy group. D. C. Jones et al. (1990) also found androgynous individuals to have more friends than those holding masculine, feminine, or undifferentiated roles.

Expressivity and self-disclosure have been shown to benefit both males' and females' same-sex friendships (e.g., Camarena et al., 1990; G. P. Jones & Dembo, 1989) and are more characteristic of men's same-sex friendships than earlier research would suggest (Inman, 1996). Similarly, Wright (in press) also cautioned our accepting the "women sacrifice activity in lieu of talk" and "men sacrifice talk in lieu of activity" dichotomy. Wright showed that dichotomizing men's and women's friendships has been based on inaccurate comparisons of frequencies and on interpretations that emphasize differences over similarities (e.g., Caldwell and Peplau, 1982, found that 57% of women preferred talk and 43% of women preferred other activities; these authors also reported a chi-square value at $p > .10$, although they interpreted this as indicating a substantial sex difference). Wright concluded that women's same-sex friendships are just as instrumental as men's, but that women's friendships are moderately more communal than are men's.

Opposite-Sex Friendships

Both men and women acknowledge that involvement in an opposite-sex friendship provides insight on the opposite sex (Sapadin, 1988). That is, a primary reason for maintaining a cross-sex friendship appears to be an increased understanding about the attitudes, beliefs, and values of members of the opposite sex.

Some research on opposite-sex friendships suggests that they are more beneficial for and regarded in higher favor by men than women (Aukett et al., 1988). Findings also suggest that men's minimized expressivity may be more central to same-sex friendships than to opposite-sex friendships. For example, Narus and Fischer (1982) found that expressivity related more to sex roles in same- than in opposite-sex friendships and that the masculine sex role related to expressivity whereas the female sex role did not.

The literature indicates that men more comfortably experience intimacy (i.e., expression of feelings) in cross-sex friendships than in same-sex friendships (e.g., Rose, 1985). Aukett et al. (1988) found that, in comparison to women, men were more likely to discuss personal problems with opposite-sex friends, and they gained more relational support and therapeutic value (i.e., empathy and intimacy) from cross-sex friendships (48%) than from same-sex friendships (10%). As well, men were more apt to cancel an engagement with a same-sex friend to accommodate an opposite-sex friend. Yet, these findings should be interpreted within the context of *similarities* between men and women and their perceived rewards for friendship. For instance, Rose found that both men and women reported that more functions are served by same- versus opposite-sex friends (e.g., acceptance, common interests, affection), although men (vs. women) reported they obtained more intimacy in opposite-sex friendships.

There are several reasons why men (vs. women) report more intimacy and support in their opposite-sex friendships compared to their same-sex friendships. First, men often feel closer to women, which is particularly beneficial during trying times (Aukett et al., 1988). As noted in the previous chapter, men more often tend to withhold expressing emotions. Yet, during times of crisis, men may seek a female friend over a male friend to discuss a problem, as they report being understood more by women (Buhrke & Fuqua, 1987) and appear to gain therapeutic value from their female friends (Aukett et al., 1988).

A second reason relates to the first: Men likely consider their opposite-sex friendships as more intimate because cross-sex involvements are more conducive to revealing personal features of the self. In particular, men may experience less homophobia when revealing self and confiding in a female friend than when sharing feelings with a male friend (Inman, 1996; Lewis, 1978). As indirect evidence of this, Snell (1989) found that men tended to reveal more of their femininity in opposite-sex friendships.

A final reason refers to the sexual aspect of opposite-sex friendships. Specifically, men tend to perceive opposite-sex relationships more sexually than women do (Abbey, 1982). Given possible sexual overtones of their interactions with women, men might consider the possible romantic evolution of an opposite-sex friendship more than women do (Rawlins, 1993). Women, on the other hand, may regard same-sex friendships more favorably over opposite-sex friendships because same-sex friendships can alleviate the possible suspicion that the opposite-sex friend entertains a sexual motive (Rose, 1985). In other words, women may question an opposite-sex friend's "true" intentions or agenda. Similarly, Bell (1981) found that men believe that they should attempt to convert opposite-sex friendships to romantic, sexual ones.

We should caution against a monolithic view of men as sexually oriented. Research has found that men's motives for maintaining opposite-sex friendships extend beyond a sexual one about 70% of the time; that is, men as well as women much more commonly value the rewards, supportiveness, and security provided by cross-sex friends in lieu of sexual interests (Messman, Canary, & Hause, 1994). In addition, Messman et al. (1994) found that some men and women have not even thought about a sexual relationship with their cross-sex friends. Morevoer, the effect for sex differences on sexual perceptions largely disappears with age, with older (middle-aged) men reporting less sexual orientations and more platonic orienta- tions toward women than do men in their 20s (Montgomery, 1987). Perhaps most critically, once cross-sex friends negotiate their friend- ships, the sexual impulses appear to subside. For example, although Rose (1985) reported that men (vs. women) were more attracted to their cross-sex friends during the initial phase of the relationship, she also reported that sexual attraction in the maintenance phase for both sexes subsides to the point where it is no different than the sexual urges experienced in same-sex friendships.

Not all research, of course, suggests that men and women clearly differ in the expression of intimacy. For example, Monsour's (1992) research outlines men's and women's self-reported behavioral indicators of intimacy in same- and opposite-sex friendships: (1) self-disclosure, (2) emotional expressiveness, (3) unconditional support, (4) physical con- tact, (5) trust, (6) activities, and (7) sexual contact. All meanings, with an exception of activities and sexual contact, were similarly reported by men and women in reference to same- and opposite-sex friendships. Regarding opposite-sex friendships only, women reported physical contact (i.e., contact that is not of a sexual nature) *more* than men did, whereas men reported emotional expressiveness and sexual contact more than women did. All other indicators of intimacy appear to be similarly perceived between the two sexes.

ROMANTIC INVOLVEMENTS

According to Hatfield (1983), one "way in which theorists agree men and women differ is in desire for intimacy" (p. 125). The literature on men, women, and intimacy in the context of romantic relationships often reports variability in how men and women approach and perceive intimacy (Prager, 1995). In this section, we first focus on research concerning relational expectations that men and women hold for romantic partners. Next we discuss date initiations by men and women.

Men's and Women's Relational Expectations

Similar to other researchers of relational expectations (e.g., L. Margolin, 1989; Matula, Huston, Grotevant, & Zamutt, 1992), Hammersla and Frease-McMahan (1990) examined university students' views on relationships and long-term goals. Results indicated that women rated relationships higher than did men, although both men and women were similar in rating goals and willingness to sacrifice goals for the relationship. Sex differences, however, appeared in men's and women's types of goals. Specifically, men placed more emphasis on physical fitness, financial success, and career than did women. Women placed more emphasis on religiosity. Overall, the few gender differences that did occur fit the traditional gender stereotypes.

Traditional stereotypes and some research suggest that women (vs. men) aspire more to marry (Inglis & Greenglass, 1989). The majority of Western men and women, however, do marry (Prager, 1995). Unfortunately, marriage and family have been associated with constant career setbacks for women and career rewards for men (cf. Chapter 5, this volume; Cooney & Uhlenberg, 1991). Matula et al. (1992) examined the association among education, finances, gender role, commitment to the dating relationship, certainty about future vocation, and views on work versus marriage as a source of life satisfaction. Results from a sample of university students indicated that the more certain an upper-division woman was about her vocational identity, the more committed she was to her dating partner. However, women who emphasized the importance of work more than marriage had more certainty about vocational identity and reported less involvement in their dating relationships. Finally, women's anticipated working after marriage was negatively associated with involvement in intimate relationships. These findings suggest that women's recognition of a career identity corresponds to commitment to their romantic relationships; but anticipating work after marriage or perceiving work after marriage as important negatively associated with commitment to the relationship.

Similarly, the clearer the vocational identity for upper-division men, the more committed they were to their relationships (Matula et al., 1992). For lower-division men, the more work was emphasized over marriage, the less involved they were in the relationship. Finally, lower-division men with more liberal gender attitudes were less clear about their vocational identity. For upper-division men, the opposite held true. These results offer an alternative to traditional roles, particularly for women. However, these results also pose possible role conflicts for women, who often juggle professional and personal commitments. Still, it appears that women temper their commitment with beliefs regarding the tenuous aspects of marriage and the importance of work.

Date Initiation

When one thinks of a traditional, heterosexual dating relationship, one often thinks of romance, commitment, and sex (e.g., "boy meets girl" scenario in which both sexes assume conventional gender roles). Research regarding men, women, and dating, however, reveals interesting findings about the dating phenomena. According to Hatfield (1983), men and women are becoming more similar versus dissimilar in their sexual experiences and preferences. However, other research indicates that men and women still adhere to their traditional gender roles when it comes to modern-day romantic relationships (e.g., Ganong & Coleman, 1992; Ickes, 1993).

The relationship between gender and dating anxiety has also been explored (e.g., Quackenbush, 1990; Robins, 1986). For example, Robins examined the relationship between gender roles and dating anxiety as well as the degree to which that relationship is generalizable across same- and opposite-sex relationships. Results revealed a positive relationship between masculinity and dating efficacy and a negative relationship between masculinity and discomfort in opposite-sex situations.

These results parallel previously cited findings that men sometimes find opposite-sex friendships more rewarding and women tend to find same-sex friendships more rewarding. Perhaps in assuming masculine roles, men comfortably take the initiative (Robins, 1986). At first glance, these results do not comport with Snell's (1989) finding that cross-sex friendships enable men to reveal more of their feminine side. One possible explanation may be that Snell's research focused on opposite-sex friendship whereas Robins's focused on opposite-sex romance. As Ickes (1993) reported, men and women seeking romance tend initially to cling to traditionally defined gender roles, and people appear to be more attracted to stereotypic features of the opposite sex (e.g., women as delicate and demure; men as strong and assertive). Over time, however, continued adherence to stereotyped expectations is negatively associated with relational quality (Ickes, 1993).

Another study on dating anxiety and gender roles provides additional support for the benefits of men's adopting the androgynous gender role. Specifically, Quackenbush (1990) examined the relationship between males' gender roles and comfort in dating and sexual situations. Men with androgynous gender roles reported the most comfort and confidence in dating and sexual situations. Conversely, men holding undifferentiated roles reported the least comfort and confidence in close, dating relationships and sexual situations. Men assuming masculine gender roles were more confident and comfortable with sex and dating than were undifferentiated men, but less comfortable than were androgynous men.

Interestingly, although the female (vs. the male) gender role should predict involvement in the relationship and romanticism, men tend to be more inclined to be affected by "love at first sight" than are women. These findings echo Z. Rubin, Peplau, and Hill's (1980) argument that men more typically buy into romantic idealism. As well, men's romantic tendencies may be related to the masculine, traditional gender role in which the man initiates and takes control of the relationship and the woman serves as the relational gatekeeper (Allgeier & Royster, 1991). Or the tendency of men more readily to adopt a romantic persona could be related to women's desire to be confident in their selection of a mate who possesses staying power and status (Trost & Alberts, in press). As romantic relationships progress from initiation to more advanced stages, men and women more frequently engage in other behaviors. The next section explores sex differences in sexual intimacy and sexuality.

SEX DIFFERENCES AND SEX

In considering the notions of "romantic relationships," "intimacy," and "sex differences," people often reference sexual intimacy (Sprecher & McKinney, 1993). In the following pages, we consider sex differences in the expression of sexual intimacy and sexuality (as a function of one's sex role identity).

Sexual Intimacy

Conclusions drawn from much of the research are often "stereotypical" in terms of what men and women supposedly seek in terms of intimacy and intimate relationships: that is, that men typically strive for sexual intimacy in romantic relationships and balk at more emotional, interdependent, nurturing closeness (Abbey, 1982; Bell, 1981), whereas women generally strive for emotional connection and interdependence while they serve as relational gatekeepers on the sexual front (e.g., Allgeier & Royster, 1991).

Several findings indicate that men and women approach the issue of sexual intimacy differently. For example, one study involving a sample of undergraduate students and a sample of recently married couples found that women prefer sexual activities that demonstrate love and intimacy whereas men prefer sexual activities primarily for the arousal component associated with them (Hatfield, Sprecher, Pillemer, Greenberger, & Wexler, 1988). Likewise, Brigman and Knox (1992) found that, of the 70% of university men and women who had engaged in sexual intercourse within the last 3 months, 67% had done so to express and share emotional intimacy. Women, however, were more likely to engage in sex to achieve emotional intimacy whereas men were more likely to engage in sex to release sexual tension.

The above findings coincide with existing research suggesting that women link sex with emotional involvement whereas men associate sex with casual, physical involvement (e.g., Abbey, 1982; Allgeier & Royster, 1991; Baldwin & Baldwin, 1990; Goodchilds & Zellman, 1984). One experiment involved a male or female subject approaching a member of the opposite sex and propositioning him/her, requesting that he/she go to the subject's apartment (Clark, 1990). Clark found that, in general, a man was more willing to go the apartment of a woman he had just met and engage in casual sex with her than the other way around.

Whether we like it or not, research supports the notion that young men typically *act* and young women typically *react* in regard to sex (Grauerholz & Serpe, 1985). Townsend (1995) addressed the stereotypical male "green light" and female "red light" behavior from an evolutionary perspective. Specifically, Townsend examined men's and women's motivation to have sex, ability to dissociate pleasure from need for investment, and emotional reactions to their engagement in low-investment sexual intercourse. Results indicated that women who engaged in low-investment sexual intercourse on their own accord often felt emotionally vulnerable and felt anxious about their partners' willingness to invest and such feelings were positively correlated with number of partners. For men, however, number of partners was negatively correlated with feeling emotionally vulnerable and feelings of anxiety due to their partners' willingness to invest. Townsend concluded that the emotions and motivations that regulate sexual arousal and attraction are sometimes dichotomous. In a word, men (vs. women) tend to be better able to avoid becoming emotionally vulnerable. One reason for this stems from women's potentially for the massive investment of pregnancy and caring for children, which men do not face (Kedrick & Trost, 1997). In other words, women carry and bear children, and then more often than men bear the responsibility for raising the children.

We believe that one cannot discuss the matter of sexual intimacy without understanding sex differences in individuals' sexuality. In our view, alternative foci of sexual activities lead to different understandings of sex as an expression of intimacy. For this reason, we develop the idea of sex differences in sexual intimacy a step further by focusing on individual differences (men vs. women) in terms of *sexuality*.

Sexuality

Do women and men possess different sexualities? The answer is inconclusive. Cultural perceptions, individual expectations, and desire may illuminate the differences hypothesized about women's and men's sexuality. Differences in sexual intimacy, if they do exist, probably stem from expectations (as discussed below).

The "cultural" perception, as indicated in the previous section, holds that women focus on feelings and men focus exclusively on sexual activity. A pressure exists for men to have frequent sex, not to confuse love with attraction, and to have sex with as many women as possible because this is their sexual nature (Hite, 1987). Women are often viewed as either "scores" or "mothers" in relation to male sexuality.

Unfortunately, not much knowledge exists about women's sexuality, probably because of the widespread assumption that women are not as sexual as men. Nin (1992) asserted that women have not made the distinction between love and sensuality. Hite's (1987) report on women and love gives credence to the notion that women make little separation between sex and affection. Many of the women's voices speak of the desire for sex and love; 83% of the women Hite surveyed wanted sex in the context of emotional involvement, whereas 13% of single women reported liking casual sex and one-night stands.

As noted earlier, men and women often report sexual intimacy as an aspect of relational intimacy (Sprecher & McKinney, 1993). Yet, reasons for intimacy and ways of being "intimate" vary for men and women (Brigman & Knox, 1992; Prager, 1995). Similarly, men's and women's views on what justifies engaging in sexual activity in dating and marital relationships may differ (L. Margolin, 1989). Specifically, whereas women often engage in sex in an effort to achieve intimacy, men often engage in sex to engage in sex (e.g., Hatfield et al., 1988).

For example, L. Margolin (1989) examined university students' ratings of partners' outside involvements in dating and marital relationships. Specifically, participants rated scenarios in which one of the dating or married partners individually participated in an outside sexual or nonsexual situation. Women participating in the study reported infidelity to be unacceptable in either dating or marital situations whereas males reported that unfaithful dating partners should be given more freedom than married partners. Considering both dating and marital relationships, women rated infidelity "very unacceptable" in both dating and marriage. Men, however, viewed infidelity in dating relationships as "moderately unacceptable" (p. 78). Men also rated marriage as more emotionally and sexually restrictive than did women, whereas women rated dating and marriage similarly.

L. Margolin's (1989) results suggest that men hold different standards for dating and marital relationships in terms of what is deemed as acceptable behavior. Specifically, the findings support the notion that men are socialized to "conquer" and to experience a variety of relationships and sexual partners rather than remain satisfied in an exclusive, monogamous relationship. Women, however, seem to discriminate less between relationship types in terms of appropriate and inappropriate sexual behavior. Overall, Margolin's results indicate that women generally hold the belief that "a romantic relationship is a romantic relationship" and what constitutes "acceptable" behavior for spouse holds for a dating partner. Such guidelines suggest that women experience more emotional attachment than men, attachment that does not discriminate relational stage. Thus, for women, alterations in relational partners or relational rules may be due to a change of heart rather than just for the sake of change. Similarly, Glass and Wright (1992) found that women are more likely to endorse love than sex as justification for an affair. The authors concluded that women are more likely to believe that love and sex are complementary and that being in love justifies sexual involvement. Men, on the other hand, have been reported to separate sex from love.

Following the sexual revolution people might presume the demise of the double standard that asserts that women "should" not be as sexually experienced as their male partners. The double standard translates into our expectations of what "natural" female and male sexuality is like. This rather essentialist stance presumes that women do not desire sex as much as men, or if they do, such desire indicates an abnormality (contrary to an idea from the previous century of a ravenous female sexuality). Research findings, however, indicate that reports of the demise may be premature.

Sprecher and McKinney (1993), after reviewing the literature, concluded with a cautionary note that the traditional double standard appears dead, but a conditional double standard still exists; that is, it is acceptable for women to have sex as long as they are involved in a committed relationship. For instance, men have different standards for dating and marriage partners. In Oliver and Sedikides (1992), participants were asked to rate the dating and marriage desirability of low- and high-permissive partners. A low-permissive male was judged by women to be the most desirable for marriage and dating. The most desirable dating partners for men, on the other hand, were women who engaged in a high level of sexual activity, though an acceptable marriage partner was a low-permissive woman. Because of such differing expectations regarding female and male sexuality, many women conceal or understate their sexual behavior (L. B. Rubin, 1990).

Sex differences in sexuality may be explained by activities related to a focus on coitus. Sexuality is usually depicted and discussed in terms of penetration (i.e., intercourse). One issue here concerns whether or not the perception of difference between women's and men's sexuality arises because sex remains defined in purely coital terms. For instance, *foreplay,* the word describing certain sexual acts such as fondling, kissing, and caressing, describes only actions that lead up to the "main event" of intercourse, rather than being considered a vital, intimate activity. Many women desire touching as much, if not more, as having intercourse itself (Sprecher & McKinney, 1993). Men may appear myopic in their focus on coitus as the central act in sexual relations. Hite (1987) stressed that "our culture's lessons to men have been so strong that few men have been able to go past them, to create their own personal sexuality, or to transcend the double standard" (p. 218).

Including a broader spectrum of activity and feelings in definitions of both women's and men's sexuality may erase some difference, such as sexual desire. The fact that sexuality does not stem only from a biological imperative but is also socially constructed should be considered when discussing differences between women and men in the arena of sexuality (see Tiefer, 1995). Ideas of what it means to be female and male characterize our sexual expectations. Much of what we consider to be "natural" sexuality is, in fact, learned behavior.

Desire for emotional attachment undoubtedly affects intimacy levels in a relationship. Individuals seeking comfort and support in a relationship likely feel "intimate" with an individual when the feelings of support or comfort are experienced (e.g., Turner, 1994). Given that individuals hold different perceptions of the same events, people may also identify "intimate" as "companionate," "passionate," "sexual," and so forth, and identify a relationship as intimate or loving when companionate, passionate, or sexual feelings are experienced with the other individual (Hecht, Marston, & Larkey,

1994). Thus, it appears to us that one's need for closeness can confound one's interpretation of what sexual expressions signify for both the relationship and one's gender role identity.

CONCLUSION

Men's and women's perceptions of and approaches to intimacy are reflected in various interaction contexts. These involve self-disclosure (e.g., Dindia & Allen, 1992), touch (e.g., Emmers & Dindia, 1995), and sexual behavior (e.g., Allgeier & Royster, 1991), in both friendship (e.g., Caldwell & Peplau, 1982; Rawlins, 1992) and romantic relationships (e.g., Prager, 1995). Such definitions of intimate behavior appear to be biased toward a feminine view of intimacy—intimacy that focuses on connection, for example, through disclosure and touch (J. J. Wood, 1993). Yet, other research shows that men and women appear to associate similar terms with intimacy.

Sex differences in the area of self-disclosure were reported: Women as a rule appear to disclose more and to use disclosure as an intimacy-related activity. However, the differences are neither consistent nor impressive. We concur with Dindia and Allen's (1992) conclusion: "The results of this meta-analysis indicate that sex differences in self-disclosure are not as large as self-disclosure theorists and researchers have suggested. It is time to stop perpetuating the myth that there are large sex differences in men's and women's self-disclosure" (p. 118).

Likewise, sex differences in touching behavior were also reported. In particular, it appears more acceptable for women to touch men in social contexts. Yet, as expressions of intimacy, sex crosses with relationship duration to affect touch: Women feel more comfortable touching later in the relationships, whereas men feel more comfortable touching in the initial stages of relational development. Women, in comparison to their male partners, report being touched more, though such differences can be traced to expectations derived from gender roles rather than actual behavior. Along these lines, we implied earlier in this chapter that presumed reasons for touching (women touch to nurture, men touch to control) represent the same stereotypical understanding of men and women and simultaneously lead to different behavioral predictions. Accordingly, it appears that finding any difference in touch could be taken as support for stereotypical thinking.

Friendships of men and women are more similarly than differently perceived. For instance, Rose (1985) found that more functions are served by same- versus opposite-sex friends (e.g., acceptance, common interests, affection), although men (vs. women) reported they obtained more intimacy in opposite-sex friendships. Although people may suspect cross-sex friends are engaging in sexual intercourse, the research suggests that a substantial majority of cross-sex friends do not and that they value their cross-sex friendships for other reasons. Wright (in press) cautions us not to focus on differences between the sexes in their friendships as the research indicates that more similarity than difference exists between the sexes in terms of how friendships function.

Although men and women tend to agree on the behavioral manifestations of intimacy more often than not, they sometimes interpret "intimacy" in different terms. Most clearly, men and women similarly engage in sexual activity in an effort to get closer to their partner (Sprecher & McKinney, 1993). But men's and women's reasons for engaging in sexual activity may not be recognized by the other. Other research suggests some variation on the general orientations that men and women have: Whereas women more than men tend to engage in sex in an effort to escalate relational intimacy, men more than women tend to engage in sex to engage in sex. Part of the reason for alternative expressions of intimacy through the medium of sex may stem from alternative understandings of sexuality in the first place (i.e., alternative foci on coitus). Likewise, women tend to perceive "close" as emotional and interdependent whereas men are more likely to perceive "close" as involving sex (e.g., Allgeier & Royster, 1991).

4

❖

Communicating Control

People in personal relationships not only experience and express intimacy, they also experience and express control (i.e., which partner influences the other). Intimacy entails interdependence, and interdependence requires coordination of actions and activities in such a way that one person tends to take the lead or both partners share leadership (Braiker & Kelley, 1979). Personal relationship scholars have long noted that how relational partners control each other affects the stability and quality of their relationships. For example, Morton, Alexander, and Altmann (1976) argued that "mutuality of control" is necessary to the viability of all personal relationships. By mutuality of control, Morton et al. refer to consensus between partners regarding who has the right to influence the other. Similarly, Kelley (1979) indicated that control issues are better decided bilaterally (i.e., by both partners) than unilaterally (i.e., one person deciding how to manage the issue without much concern for consensus) in terms of coordinating actions ("behavioral control") and making decisions about future outcomes ("fate control").

In this chapter we examine how sex differences in control and power/dominance are exercised in personal relationships in partners' influence strategies, conflict communication, conversational behaviors, and relational maintenance strategies (see also Kalbfleisch & Cody, 1995, for reviews). We confine ourselves to research concerning normative, nonviolent methods of conveying power, though the research on physical and psychological aggression represents an important domain of behavior that may vary according to sex differences (Eagly & Steffen, 1986; Marshall, 1994; Spitzberg, 1997). Nor do we examine other contexts, for example, how leaders emerge in group discussions (for a review, see Aries, 1996).

POWER AND POWERFUL BEHAVIOR

Definitions of *power* typically have referenced resources that an individual possesses (Felmlee, 1994; McDonald, 1980). That is, power resides in the actual resources an individual can wield to influence others, and one's latitude of influence depends on one's power bases in operation. Researchers explicitly or implicitly adopting a view of power as an "individual resource" may presume that men (vs. women) hold more power given the relative number and type of resources that men possess (e.g., income, social status, physical strength, etc.).

A less commonly used "relational definition" view of power refers to how both partners define their influence potential to each other (Berger, 1994). Thus, actual or objectively defined resources are not required for one to influence the partner. Instead, one's power bases that are both *perceived* and *respected* by the partner carry more weight in determining one's selection and enactment of influence strategies. For example, the "principle of least interest" indicates that the person who feels less dependent on the other holds more power. People compose this principle largely as a function of how important the relationship is to each person, and little objective basis for the principle may exist.

A "communicative" view of power refers to how communication itself determines the power relationship between partners. As McDonald (1980) suggested, following his review of the literature, one's resources are filtered by one's interpersonal skills and competence. Accordingly, interactions between people indicate each person's relative power over the other. For example, some scholars assume that feminine forms of communicating—such as use of hedges and tag questions—reflect a person's submissiveness to the partner (for a review, see Mulac & Bradac, 1995). Other communicative accomplishments of power include use of interruptions, one-up versus one-down messages, and nonverbal behaviors.

In our view, power can originate from individual resources and attributions regarding such resources, relational definitions, and/or communicative accomplishments. Individuals undoubtedly vary in their personal as well as interpersonal resources. Accordingly, people can rely on power bases that might exist in fact, in perception, and/or in their communicative ability to influence others. The combination of these orientations helps explain how someone can intimidate without appearing intimidating and how a person can appear quite intimidating to someone who in fact enjoys more power resources. Although a fully articulated model of power remains outside the purview of this project, we nevertheless want to underscore that power may not be restricted to one location. Instead, a synthesis of power approaches enlarges the scope of our exploration of sex differences in controlling behavior as an individual, relational, and communicated factor. In other words, sex and gender differences in how partners control each other can be revealed in the way that power is communicated as much as (or even more than) the way it might be presumed to stem from social status indicators and attributions of resources.

SEX DIFFERENCES IN POWER STRATEGIES

Characterizing Power Strategies

Power (or influence) strategies refer to general behavioral approaches one takes with the partner in order to gain compliance from the partner. By extension, *power tactics* refer to specific communication behaviors that compose and institute one's general strategic orientation during interaction. In other words, power tactics operationally define one's power strategy.

Researchers have provided underlying dimensions of communication strategies and tactics. One popular dimension distinguishes strategies and tactics on their *directness* (e.g., Falbo & Peplau, 1980; Sillars & Wilmot, 1994; or a similar dimension like "activeness," van de Vliert & Euwema, 1994). The directness dimension references behaviors that first are quite overt, direct, responsive, and active versus behaviors that are covert, indirect, unresponsive, and inactive. Researchers also have stressed some feature of *valence,* or the positive–negative implications the message conveys either as a reflection of the social actor's emotional state or opinion of the partner. Falbo and Peplau's (1980) *unilateral–bilateral* dimension, for example, differentiates power strategies on the basis of whether the partner's response matters (e.g., withdrawal vs. bargaining). van de Vliert and Euwema's (1994) *disagreeableness* dimension indicates how unpleasant and restraining the strategy appears to be.

Using the dimensions of directness and valence, we might predict sex differences generally in the use of various power and influence strategies and tactics. From the stereotypic view (which we hold is general but inaccurate) men are viewed as instrumental and dominant. Accordingly, one would anticipate that men (vs. women) engage in more direct and negative influence behaviors (Falbo & Peplau, 1980; Sagrestano, 1992). On the other hand, given the stereotypic view (again, general but inaccurate) of women as communal, one might presuppose that women (vs. men) are more indirect and positive in their use of power behavior. As the literature shows, people in close involvements present a more complex picture of men's and women's power strategies.

The Use of Power Strategies

Several studies have directly examined whether men or women act in more powerful ways to persuade their partners. In an influential study on the topic, Falbo and Peplau (1980) hypothesized, "Thus it may be that men's greater power in relationships is the basis for sex differences in power strategies used in intimate relationships" (p. 619). Falbo and Peplau's rationale for men's greater power appears to derive from traditional gender roles (p. 618), though they also recognized that perceptions of power also can affect power strategies used in close involvements (p. 619). Falbo and Peplau examined essays of heterosexual and homosexual university students regarding how they influenced a present or past romantic partner. Contrary to what the authors predicted based on sex role stereotypes, heterosexual men reported a greater reliance on bilateral and direct power tactics than women did, and heterosexual women indicated that they used *more* unilateral and indirect strategies. Falbo and Peplau also reported that gay men did not differ from lesbians in the use of power strategies.

Falbo and Peplau (1980) interpreted these findings as indicating that straight men use bilateral strategies from their position of strength, whereas women do not believe they can influence their partner and therefore engage in unilateral behaviors from a relative position of weakness that anticipates a partner's resistance. However, Falbo and Peplau reported the following examples, offered by female participants, to support their interpretation: " 'If what I want to do is more important and we can do it together, we do it, and vice versa. If not, we do whatever we want to do separately.' Another woman wrote, 'I'm straightforward. If he doesn't want to do what I want to do, I usually do it without him!' " (p. 627). We do not see how such behaviors reflect a position of weakness. Indeed, Falbo and Peplau's interpretation adheres to the dominance model they used initially as a frame of reference. Other research has shown that dating couples have equal power and that they perceive their relationships as more or less equal in terms of power (Felmlee, 1994; cf. Sprecher, 1985).

In an extension of Falbo and Peplau (1980), Sagrestano (1992) examined student participant reports of what they would say in three hypothetical situations involving a friend. Using ratings, rankings, and essays, Sagrestano found that men and women "used" identical messages. Both men and women reported a greater reliance on bilateral strategies when in equal relationships. Such behaviors included use of persuasion, reasoning, asking, discussing, and persistence. Although expectations based on stereotypes indicate that men rely more on power strategies, "when women were placed in positions of power they were just as likely to use these strategies as were men, which indicates that power differences had a more profound effect than did [sex] on the choice of strategies used by individuals" (p. 493).

Other research suggests that, within dating relationships, women attempt to exert more control than do men. Stets (1993) hypothesized the following: "Men's less frequent perspective taking may have the effect of increasing conflict in relationships and generating the feeling that situations are out of their control.

Controlling others would help counterbalance the sense of diminished control" (p. 677). In short, Stets hypothesized greater control efforts by men (vs. women). Stets then interviewed men and women in dating, seriously dating, and engaged relationships over the phone to assess their perspective taking, controlling behaviors, and conflict issues. Controlling behaviors included such actions as keeping tabs on the partner, regulating what the partner does, imposing one's will on the partner, and the like. Contrary to her hypothesis, Stets found that *women* (vs. men) controlled their dating partners more. Nor did Stets find any sex differences in perspective-taking. In interpreting these results, Stets suggested that women may feel threatened because their control is limited to love relationships or that men may have underreported their more frequent controlling behaviors.

Manipulation Tactics

The effects due to sex on manipulation behavior are not uniform. Buss, Gomes, Higgins, and Lauterbach (1987) asked couples who had been dating for at least 6 months to indicate the likelihood that they as well as their partner would engage in each of six manipulation tactics (i.e., reason, regression, coercion, charm, debasement, and silent treatment). Only 2 of 35 behaviors differed between men and women, and only one tactic was associated with self-reported power. Men and women alike preferred using reason, then charm, regression, coercion, silent treatment, and debasement. And of these tactics, only regression was associated with women's power; women's self-reported power was *positively* associated with women's use of regression. Considering that regression reflects a weak position, this finding appears anomalous to the view that women use manipulation from a position of weakness.

Sex differences in the use of "strong" versus "weak" tactics were explored by Howard, Blumstein, and Schwartz (1986). Strong strategies were *bullying* (threats, insults, ridicule, violence) and *autocracy* (insistence, claims of greater knowledge, assertions of authority); weak strategies were indirect *manipulation* (dropped hints, flattery, persuasion, references to past favors) and the more direct *supplication* (pleading, crying, acting ill or helpless). Howard et al. also referred to "neutral" strategies of *disengagement* (sulking, guilt-tripping, leaving the scene) and *bargaining* (reasoning with, compromises, offering trade-offs). Howard and colleagues found that sex differences combined with other indicators of relational power to affect the perception of partner's weak tactics (i.e., manipulation and supplication). More specifically, men reported that their partners were more likely to use manipulation and supplication, though the effect sizes were very weak (*r*'s = .19 and .11, respectively, accounting for less than 2% of the variance).

Howard et al. (1986) also found some intriguing interaction effects that help clarify the role of sex in predicting weak tactics. The authors reported that women's employment affected variation in perception of their influence behaviors. Specifically, heterosexual women who were not employed were said to engage more in supplication (beta = .26), and they were perceived as using the strong strategies of bullying (beta = .20) and autocracy (beta = .30); male partners of women who stay at home were more likely than their male counterparts to be perceived as using the weak strategy of manipulation (beta = −.26). In addition, the presence of children appears to increase the likelihood of using weaker strategies, among both lesbian and heterosexual women. Finally, increased dependence on the partner was positively correlated with use of supplication among heterosexual men and women, and lesbian women, and the use of manipulation among heterosexual women and homosexual men. The authors interpreted these data to indicate that the desire to maintain the relationship over time promotes the use of weaker tactics (vs. bullying or autocracy), but that sex and gender role differences do not dramatically affect the use of weak tactics.

In short, although women appear to use a wider variety of indirect and negative influence behaviors, the effect sizes due to sex differences are small. Some research has shown that men and women largely prefer the same strategies. Other research shows that women appear to use more unilateral and controlling behaviors in romantic relationships, contrary to initial expectations that rely on stereotypic conceptions of men and women (Falbo & Peplau, 1980; Stets, 1993).

What happens when men and women attempt to influence each other and their attempts are met with resistance? This question has been addressed in research examining conflict interactions of men and women.

SEX DIFFERENCES IN MANAGING INTERPERSONAL CONFLICT

Confronting the Stereotype, Again

As indicated in Chapter 1, stereotypic understandings of men and women communicating indicate that selection and use of conflict behaviors are guided by instrumental concerns for men and by communal concerns for women. Accordingly, women would enact more positive and direct conflict behaviors, such as offering information, describing the problem, soliciting disclosure, and compromising; men would rely on competitive behaviors, including personal criticism, blaming, and withdrawal. In this section, we consult some of the research to uncover the extent to which these stereotypic predictions hold.

The tendency to report behaviors that comport with conventional expectations probably explains why self-report more than observational studies find support for hypotheses based on stereotypes. For example, in a meta-analysis of 35 studies on conflict styles, Gayle, Preiss, and Allen (1994) reported that men are more likely to use competitive tactics and women are more likely to use compromising tactics with men. Unfortunately, virtually all of their sample studies relied on self-reported data. As Burggraf and Sillars (1987) documented, self-reported studies of conflict appear biased toward sex stereotypes, whereas observational analyses of actual interaction resist such biases. Moreover, the observational studies provide more specific records of interaction data; self-reports better reflect beliefs, attitudes, intentions, and impressions. As Markman and Notarius (1987) noted, "Perhaps the most salient factor mandating observational research is the inability of interactants to describe the ongoing behavioral process, that is, contemporary patterns of interaction" (p. 331). As with other research on sex differences in communication, self-reported sex differences outweigh observed sex differences (Fisher, 1983). In other words, and especially when sampling college students considering hypothetical scenarios, self-reported studies reflect more stereotypical behavior than what researchers have observed when assessing personal relationships of adults of all ages (Markman, Silvern, Clements, & Kraft-Hanak, 1993).

Women Confront, Men Discuss or Avoid

In general, more similarities than differences characterize men's and women's conflict management behavior; evidence from both survey and observational analyses show that sex similarities outweigh sex differences (for a review, see Cupach & Canary, 1995). For example, G. Margolin and Wampold (1981) highlighted several sex differences: wives engaged in more smiling and laughter, complaining, and criticizing, whereas husbands presented more excuses. Also, distressed husbands appeared more withdrawn (i.e., men showed less "tracking" of events). However, husbands and wives engaged in most conflict behaviors in a similar manner; spouses did not differ on 75% of the codes, including the important categories of problem solving, positive verbal comments, negative verbal comments, and negative nonverbal behaviors.

In addition, research has found the opposite of what one might hypothesize from a stereotypic understanding of men and women. For example, Canary, Cunningham, and Cody (1988), relying on the stereotype of women as communal, hypothesized that women would show more cooperative behavior to accomplish relational development and maintenance goals. However, Canary et al. found the opposite of this prediction—women (vs. men) tended to report using competitive tactics in conflicts regarding relational development and maintenance issues.

In a direct test of the hypothesis that conflict behavior follows sex stereotypes, Cupach and Canary (1995) surveyed over 100 married couples at two different times to assess their recent use of *integrative* (i.e., cooperative and direct tactics), *distributive* (i.e., competitive and direct tactics), and *avoidance* (i.e., indirect tactics) strategies. The only significant difference was that wives reported using *more* distributive tactics at both points in time, although men reported slightly higher use of integrative and avoidance tactics. Perhaps more intriguing was our finding that wives' ratings of their spouses' competence were strongly tied to the perception that the husband used distributive or avoidant behaviors, whereas husbands' ratings of wives' competence was tied to the perception that the wife was integrative. In other words, wives appeared to rely more on the husbands' negativity when judging his behavior, though the wives (vs. husbands) reported greater use of negative messages. On the contrary, husbands relied more on assessments of wife positivity, though husbands (vs. wives) self-reported more positive behavior.

In a classic observational study, Raush, Barry, Hertel, and Swain (1974) illustrated that couples variously responded to each other in terms of six conflict behaviors: *cognitive* acts, which are neutral behaviors, suggestions, and rational statements; *resolving* tactics, which include behaviors aimed at reducing tensions and at reaching a satisfactory outcome; *reconciling* acts, which attempt to bring partners together on an emotional level; *appealing* messages, which include attempts to get the partner to grant one's needs and wants; *rejecting* acts, which reveal a "cold or nasty" disavowal of the partner or the partner's ideas; and *coercive or personal attacks,* which attempt to force compliance (e.g., through use of guilt or ridicule of one's partner) (pp. 115, 214–233). Raush and colleagues found some sex role asymmetry in conflict management behaviors. More precisely, wives tended to be more coercive and appealing, whereas husbands tended to be more reconciling and resolution-minded; and this asymmetry in sex role behavior was most pronounced in dissatisfied relationships (pp. 138–174).

The above findings do not support traditional sex roles. Yet, these findings are entirely consistent with much of the literature in personal relationships. Following their review of the literature and report of original studies, Schaap, Buunk, and Kerkstra (1988) concluded, "All in all we think that self-report and observational research supports the following statements. Women tend to be more emotional and show more negative affect, while men are inclined to be more rational and withdrawn" (p. 236). For example, in an examination of verbal conflict tactics, Fitzpatrick and Winke (1979) did not find any main sex effects for the communicator or the recipients (i.e., men and women tended to use and perceive conflict tactics similarly). However, in contrasts regarding same-sex friendships, men were more likely to use nonnegotiation tactics (e.g., refuse to discuss until other gives in), whereas women preferred the use of personal rejection (e.g., act cold until the other gives in), empathic understanding (e.g., hold mutual talks), and emotional appeals (e.g., appeal to the person's love [or] demonstrate anger). In an examination of nonverbal behaviors, Noller (1982) found that wives use more negative nonverbal behaviors (e.g., frowns, scowls, angry tones) than did their husbands. In addition, wives' (vs.

husbands') affective messages were more inconsistent (e.g., wives smiled more when offering negative comments).

Granted, findings from research involving acquaintances and strangers support the stereotype of the dominant male in social situations, expressing anger and the like, and women appear to accommodate to and compromise with men (Aries, 1996; Chapter 2, this volume). But the research clearly shows that, over time and in *familiar* situations and personal relationships, women (vs. men) demonstrate more assertiveness and competitiveness (a phenomenon also found in organizations; Putnam & Wilson, 1982).

Women's (vs. men's) greater use of competitive, negative conflict behavior in personal relationships is moderated by several other factors. First, and importantly, use of negative behavior is strongly influenced by the partner's immediately preceding behavior. For instance, Burggraf and Sillars (1987) compared the effects of sex to the effects of the spouse's preceding communication behavior. In two observational studies, the partner's antecedent conflict behavior was a stronger predictor than one's sex of one's conflict behavior. Conflict management behaviors were typically reciprocated by both spouses, overriding the effects due to sex. Burggraf and Sillars concluded that the effects due to communicator sex were "dwarfed" by effects due to interaction and couple type.

Second, and specific to the issue of negative strategy use, reviews of the research show that dissatisfied couples in particular engage in rigid sequences of negative affect (Gottman, 1994; Sillars & Wilmot, 1994). In other words, people in dissatisfied marriages are more likely than their satisfied counterparts to reciprocate negative messages. For example, Ting-Toomey (1983) found that dissatisfied couples frequently enacted 10 turns of attack–defend messages! Noller, Feeney, Bonnell, and Callan (1994) found that negativity was associated with a decline in satisfaction over time. Satisfied spouses were less likely to engage in manipulation, threats, and demand–withdrawal patterns (see below). Accordingly, one cannot compare women's conflict behavior to men's without considering the quality of relationships under investigation.

Third, it appears that couple behavior varies according to occupation status (occupation status defined according to the "main wage earner's category"). For example, Krokoff, Gottman, and Roy (1988) found that blue collar men engaged in more negative conflict behavior than did white-collar men. Additionally, the authors reported a satisfaction by occupation interaction effect involving women: dissatisfied white-collar women enacted more negative affect compared to dissatisfied blue-collar women. The authors interpreted these findings as indicating that economic stress prompts men to vent more negative feelings. In addition, Krokoff et al. argued that dissatisfied blue-collar women do not approach the husband in part because their comparisons with other women leave them feeling relatively well-off; thus, blue-collar women feel more fortunate than do white-collar women, who expect more.

Finally, the person who wants to change the status quo is more likely to confront the partner, regardless of sex. The person who does the confronting would more likely engage in competitive, negative messages, such as demands, negative mind reading, prescriptions, and the like. This final moderating factor is nicely illustrated in research concerning the "demand–withdrawal" pattern of interaction.

The Demand–Withdrawal Pattern

In the "demand–withdrawal" pattern, men respond to women's attempts to discuss relational problems with avoidance, which stems from men's instrumentality and lack of experience at managing relational events; women, who want to increase their connection to their spouses, actively pursue their partner to engage in discussions about relational problems. However, as one might suspect, the observed sex differences do not reveal what one might anticipate.

In two studies, Markman et al. (1993) examined (1) observations of actual interaction and (2) self-reported complaints of marital partner withdrawal and demands (which they term "withdrawal" and "pursuit"). In the study of actual interaction, Markman et al. reported only one sex difference: women showed more attentive behaviors than did men. They did not find any evidence supporting the demand–withdrawal pattern. But in the second study, which examined self-reported complaints, men complained more about their partners' confrontation behavior, but women did not complain more than men about their partner's withdrawal behavior. Indeed, a crossed interaction effect showed that some men complain more than women about partner withdrawal. Nevertheless, the main effect regarding men's complaints of being confronted does provide some support for the demand–withdrawal hypothesis. However, this hypothesis was supported only for self-reported data, which Markman and colleagues emphasized in their conclusion: "In either case, the present results add to other findings that *when couples are actually observed, fewer {sex} differences emerge than indicated by their self-reports*" (p. 120, emphasis in original).

Christensen and Heavey (1990; see also Heavey, Layne, & Christensen, 1993; Kleintob & Smith, 1996; Sagrestano, Christensen, & Heavey, in press) tested two explanations for the demand–withdrawal pattern using self-report and observational data. The "individual difference" explanation leaned heavily on the stereotypic conceptions of women as communal and of men as instrumental. Women approach men and men avoid women given these differing orientations. The "structural" explanation concerned the asymmetry involved with the issue under discussion. More precisely, the person who wants the partner's compliance in order to achieve his/her own goals more likely needs to "confront" the partner. In many instances, this would involve the person who is less equitably treated to approach the partner for help (e.g., in raising a child; Christensen & Heavey, 1990). But the partner who did not require the other's help to achieve his/her goals more likely avoids the spouse. Withdrawal thus functions as a power strategy to sustain the status quo. Because men tend to experience greater benefits in marriage, they might avoid their partner to maintain those benefits (e.g., meals, a clean home, affection; Sagrestano et al., in press).

The results from this line of research are consistent and clear— the person who depends on the partner and wants to change the status quo is more likely to confront the partner, regardless of sex. However, when spouses discuss the woman's issue, the demand– withdrawal effect is more dramatic than when parties discuss the man's issue. As Sagrestano et al. (in press) concluded, this greater polarization between men and women when discussing the woman's issue of concern may reflect *both* a social structural effect (as a pattern that has developed over time) and an individual difference effect (differences in relational expectations stemming from one's sex role). Regardless, and due to the higher-ordered crossed interaction effect, one should not interpret sex role main effects apart from a consideration of whose topic is being discussed.

Explanations for Women's Negative Messages

The general tendency for women in close involvements to engage in more negative interaction and for men to shy away from such messages might be counterintuitive to most readers. In addition, the research reported in Chapter 2 indicates that men appear to experience somewhat more (not less) anger than women do, though the sexes are far more similar than different in their expression of anger. For many people, finding that women communicate with more negativity in their personal relationships is not only counterintuitive but radically invalid, given a presumed power differential that men appear to hold in the larger social realm (Felmlee, 1994; Tannen, 1990). Naturally, some people might insist that more evidence is needed before dismissing the idea that women in fact act in a manner consistent with the stereotype of women as a caring and nurturing group of people.

Several explanations have been offered for women's greater confrontation in personal relationships. In the following sections, we summarize five alternative, though neither comprehensive nor incompatible, explanations: (1) inequity in marriage, (2) Gottman and Levenson's physiological explanation, (3) development of influence activities, (4) gender role identification, and (5) Fitzpatrick's marital typology.

Inequity in Marriage

One explanation for the demand–withdrawal pattern involves an assessment of who is inequitably treated. Christensen and Heavey (1990) indicated that equity could explain the demand–withdrawal pattern: The person who was inequitably treated would be more likely to demand a change in the partner's behavior. Given that wives (vs. husbands) tend to report being less equitably treated (VanYperen & Buunk, 1990), we can understand how more women then men engage in confrontational behavior.

Along these lines, Falbo and Peplau (1980) found that a desire for equality of power within intimate relationships correlated positively and strongly with use of unilateral power tactics ($r^2 = .76$), whereas those who did not emphasize equality more likely reported they had used bilateral strategies. And women (vs. men) reported a greater desire for equality in their close involvements. It appears that partners who seek equality may feel underbenefited—that is, they obtain fewer rewards relative to inputs than do their partners. Accordingly, women would more likely be the ones to confront the partner within the negative emotions, such as sadness or anger, that accompany being inequitably treated (Sprecher, 1986).

Physiological Explanation

Gottman and Levenson's view of sex differences in marriage relies on explaining physiological reactions that husbands and wives have during conflict (Gottman, 1994; Gottman & Levenson, 1988; Levenson, Carstensen, & Gottman, 1994; Levenson & Gottman, 1983, 1985). Negative physiology is assumed to accompany negative interaction behavior. More precisely, these researchers have found that men display more negative physiological arousal arising when participating in conflict issue discussions. When discussing important problematic issues during conflict, people become negatively "charged," which is seen in faster heart rates, pulse transmission time, skin conductance levels, and somatic activity. In addition, men require longer periods of time to recover from this physiological "flooding," and husbands are more aware of their own physiological flooding than their wives are of their own.

This physiological explanation of sex differences holds that men resist discussions due to the unpleasantness arising from such discussions, whereas women (who ignore it or who experience less arousal) more readily confront their male partners (see Gottman, 1994, for a complete account). Such confrontations can lead to an imbalance in the way that couples manage conflict, where "balance" refers to the number of positive to negative statements; satisfied couples appear to have close to a 5:1 ratio (a balanced state) and dissatisfied couples experience a 1:1 ratio (an imbalanced state). The increasingly negative behaviors of complaining/criticizing, showing contempt, being defensive, and stonewalling appear to begin a "cascade" of negative affect. As indicated, men should respond with flight reactions to flooding, and several studies have supported this expectation (Gottman, 1994, for a review). Women are more likely to suffer the consequences of negative physiological arousal, which they ignore when seeking to discuss conflictual issues (Levenson et al., 1994).

As an illustration, Gottman and Krokoff (1989) videotaped

married couples as they discussed conflict issues. Gottman and Krokoff found that conflict engagement and expression of anger were negatively associated with current relational satisfaction, but these negative behaviors were associated with increases in relational satisfaction measured 3 years later. More specifically, wives' use of contempt and anger was negatively associated with concurrent marital satisfaction for both partners, but positively associated with a change in marital satisfaction for the wives. The authors interpreted these findings as indicating that husbands should not avoid their wives or whine; rather, husbands were advised to engage their wives so as to maintain the relationship over time.

Developmental Differences

Some research in developmental psychology provides an alternative reason why men might not affected by women's verbal persuasion attempts: Men's power has emerged as a function of their physical development, but not as a result of their refined communication strategies.

In reviewing research on sex segregation, where boys and girls play in groups of their own sexes, Maccoby (1988) indicated that boys learn to influence each other primarily through rough play, whereas girls rely more on verbal messages to get their way. In addition, boys acquire dominant positions in mixed-sex play groups and girls' attempts to gain influence do not prove effective. Girls' failure to adopt alternative influence techniques may serve to perpetuate sex segregation through childhood. As Maccoby argued:

> It is reasonable to assume that, in any relationship that is freely entered into by both parties, the relationship is more likely to be continued over time and be satisfactory to both parties if each can influence the behavior of the other. If girls develop influence styles that are ineffective with boys, this becomes a reason for avoiding interaction with them. It would also be a reason for girls to seek out situations in which their influence styles *would* work with boys—situations in which they might more easily hold their own in any conflicts over access to desired resources. (p. 758)

Thus, men's documented withdrawal might have its genesis in early play and may emerge as they grow older and as girls begin to adopt more effective influence styles. In this light, we can see how young boys come to appreciate a power that resides in an active, physical world; and later, as men, they rely more on physical withdrawal as one means of coping with challenges. But women (vs. men) rely more on language—verbal and nonverbal—to influence others, to the extent that as young girls they polish their communicative skills in managing personal problems. Accordingly, women tend to use a wider array of communication strategies, including negative messages, when confronting their partners.

Gender Role Identification

As indicated in Chapter 1, people can vary in the extent to which they adhere to masculine and feminine gender roles (Bem, 1981). If women believe that it is their responsibility, obligation, or even duty to maintain the relationship, then they would more likely confront the partner on important relationship issues.

Ickes's (1993) review of traditional stereotypes in close involvements shows that men and women appear to be attracted initially to those who adhere to the conventional stereotypes. However, continued adherence to stereotypical behaviors reduces one's liking for the partner. This implies that people need to alter expectations for an ideal "man" or "woman" to a more circumspect conception of gender-relevant behavior in close relationships, lest they encounter the "fundamental paradox" Ickes mentioned: traditionally masculine men and traditionally feminine women over time suffer dissatisfying relationships. In a related manner, Baucom, Notarius, Burnett, and Haefner (1990) reported a study (pp. 160–162) wherein higher levels of masculinity *and* femininity for *both* husbands and wives positively associated with dyadic adjustment (i.e., cohesion, affection, etc.). But Baucom et al. reported that being married to an undifferentiated partner (i.e., a person without either a masculine or feminine gender role orientation) was associated with lack of dyadic adjustment. These studies are not uniform in their findings; yet, they leave a combined impression that people who eschew stereotypical gender roles appear to enjoy more satisfying personal relationships.

In a study that directly examined conflict and gender role identification, Sayers and Baucom (1991) found that, among women only, femininity positively correlated with negative conflict behaviors (i.e., blame and invalidation, from the Marital Interaction Coding System; $r = .27$) and with indices of perpetuating negative sequences (r's = .31–.37). In addition, feminine women *and* men were more likely to reciprocate negative affect; that is, feminine women and men tended to terminate fewer negative sequences than did their counterparts (r's = .31 and .33, for women and men, respectively). Finally, and (again) counter to stereotypic assumptions, masculinity in women inversely correlated with negative conflict behaviors. Sayers and Baucom interpreted these findings in light of other research that shows that couples might benefit from negative emotion (e.g., displays of anger; Gottman & Krokoff, 1989): "Spouses with higher levels of femininity may be more likely to ensure that important conflictual issues are dealt with by the couple, thus increasing the chances that over time the couple will resolve these problems" (Sayers & Baucom, 1991, p. 646). However, the fact that the couples in this study were selected because they had sought marital therapy suggests that these couples had not addressed all their issues effectively with negative messages. Most research suggests that reciprocation of negative affect is detrimental to satisfaction and stability in all types of personal relationships (for a review, see Canary et al., 1995).

Marital Types

A fifth explanation concerns how men and women who adhere to alternative relational schemas might enact different gender roles. As mentioned in Chapter 1, Fitzpatrick and colleagues (e.g., Fitzpatrick, 1988a, 1988b; Witteman & Fitzpatrick, 1986) have provided convincing evidence that marriage in the latter half of the 20th century is composed of alternative types. Traditionals espouse conventional gender role beliefs, enjoy high interdependence and little personal space, and safeguard stability more than satisfaction. Independents hold egalitarian beliefs and values, desire psychological connection as well as periodic autonomy, and desire to negotiate almost everything. Separates appear to be "emotionally divorced" and rely on marriage as a way to maintain a traditional ideology without affective interdependence. Mixed couples represent a blend of marriage prototypes, where partners adhere to different marriage models. The most prevalent Mixed group is an important one for our analysis—the Separate husband and Traditional wife.

This corpus of research (Fitzpatrick, 1988a, 1988b; Witteman & Fitzpatrick, 1986) shows that both Traditional men and Traditional women appear to use relatively positive tactics; references to relationship expectations, minimal confrontation over minor issues but direct refutation in significant disagreements (i.e., counterargument), and validation and "contract" sequences (e.g., husband offers information, wife agrees). Independents, who see their partners partially in terms of their own needs and goals, actively engage each other in conflict, appear competitive even over minor issues, and exchange information and reasons for compliance. In addition, Independents are dissatisfied when their partners use avoidance as a conflict or influence strategy. Separates, who avoid interdependence, withdraw when confronted about their opinions or indirect comments, limit each other's expression of emotion, and facilitate compliance by acquiescing early.

Based on observations of couples' conflict behaviors, Gottman (1994) identified three functional and two dysfunctional couple types. According to Gottman, the three functional types resemble Fitzpatrick's types. First, *validating couples* look like Traditional couples in their emotional connection but neutral affect in managing conflict. Next, *volatile couples* resemble Independents in their engagement of each other over many issues. Finally, *conflict minimizers* look like Separates in their emotional distance. Gottman indicated that the other marital types appear dysfunctional in their reliance on defensiveness, withdrawal, and contempt. These dysfunctional couples could be represented in Fitzpatrick's Mixed types (i.e., couples that have combinations of pure types). The most common Mixed couple type contains a Traditional wife and a Separate husband (Fitzpatrick, 1988a).

It would appear that definitive sex differences would arise in the conventional Separate and Traditional marriages, and the clearest sex differences would emerge in the Traditional/Separate mixed type. In this last marriage type, the woman seeks connection with her husband, wants to plan for greater interdependence, and attempts to maintain conventional gender roles (with her viewing the marriage as primary over her own goals). However, the Separate husband seeks autonomy, safeguards his feelings, and avoids confrontation. Accordingly, the relational schemata in place for Separate/Traditional couples invite the enactment of the demand–withdrawal pattern.

DISPLAYS OF CONTROL
IN CONVERSATIONAL BEHAVIORS

People often assume that men and women control conversations differently. Sex differences in conversational control might reflect men's greater social power and status, according to the "dominance" perspective, which has been most widely used in the examination of sex differences in conversational behavior. Several subclasses of behavior indicate who enjoys a dominant orientation, and we review four of these: nonverbal controlling behaviors, style convergence in conversation, efforts expended to maintain the conversation, and interruptions.

Nonverbal Control

Relying on a "male dominance" perspective, Henley (1977) compared men and women in terms of how nonverbal communication conveys differences in status. Henley concluded her review with a summary that illustrated the "gestures of power and privilege" that men have over women. Table 4.1 presents those features of Henley's summary. As Table 4.1 shows, Henley's summary strongly supports her thesis that men enjoy the power to act with a wider latitude of behavior. However, women are constrained in the area of power (prerogative to touch, etc.) but are expected to engage in relationally promoting ways (such as disclosing, smiling, and showing emotion).

The presumption that touch and other behaviors represent power has been questioned, however. Most notably, Hall (1984) pointed out that the use of touch by men cannot be taken for granted. As Hall stated:

> When male-to-female touch asymmetry is found, there is a great need to try to document when, where, and in what relationship it occurs, and whether it is limited to certain kinds of touches. And when male-to-female asymmetry is documented, it is also unwarranted to *assume* that it is due to status discrepancy between the sexes, as some authors seem to do. . . . One possibility, supported by the touch-response literature, is that women enjoy being touched and that men, in touching them, are merely recognizing this fact. Indeed, men may respond to some subtle eliciting cue. Women's

greater appreciation of touch could, of course, have a connection to their lower status, but, if so, status has only an indirect effect on touch asymmetry. (p. 118)

Besides touching, dominance can be conveyed through gaze. Several researchers have examined sex differences in "visual dominance," or the ratio of the following: amount of eye contact while speaking divided by amount of eye contact while listening. Thus, making eye contact when one speaks but not when one listens is said to represent dominant behavior. As one might expect, sex differences in visual dominance are moderated by the task at hand and the person's competence at accomplishing the task. For example, Dovido, Ellyson, Keating, Heltman, and Brown (1988) found that, in general, men (vs. women) had higher ratios of visual dominance. However, this finding was altered by the person's expertise and ability to reward the partner. As Dovido et al. reported, "Consistent with expectation states theory, men and women high in expertise or [power to grant rewards] in our research displayed equivalent levels of looking while speaking and looking while listening (i.e., a high visual dominance ratio)" (p. 239). In addition, men engaged in greater dominance when the topic at

TABLE 4.1. Henley's (1977) Comparisons and Contrasts of Sex Differences in Interaction

	Between status equals		Between nonequals		Between sexes	
	Intimate	Nonintimate	Used by superior	Used by subordinate	Used by men	Used by women
Demeanor	Informal	Circumspect	Informal	Circumspect	Informal	Circumspect
Posture	Relaxed	Tense	Relaxed	Tense	Relaxed	Tense
Personal space	Closeness	Distance	Closeness (option)	Distance	Closeness	Distance
Touching	Touch	Don't touch	Touch (option)	Don't touch	Touch	Don't touch
Eye contact	Establish	Avoid	Stare, ignore	Avert eyes, watch	Stare, ignore	Avert eyes, watch
Emotional expression	Show	Hide	Hide	Show	Hide	Show
Self-disclose	Disclose	Don't disclose	Don't disclose	Disclosure	Don't disclose	Disclose

Note. Adapted from Henley (1977). Included here are those behaviors that were not qualified with the statement "Behavior not known" (p. 181). Copyright 1977 by Prentice-Hall. Adapted by permission.

hand was a masculine one, and women engaged in greater dominance when the topic was a feminine one.

Similarly, W. Wood and Karten (1986) found that expertise in a task moderated the effects of sex on perceived competence and task-relevant behavior. In general, men were perceived as more competent. Yet, no sex differences were found in "status-specified" conditions (i.e., when expertise was manipulated): Relative to low status participants, high status people engaged in less friendly social behavior, spoke more frequently, used more active and passive task-related behavior, and enacted more negative social behavior. The authors concluded that sex's "lack of impact in the status-specified conditions indicates that the most weight or importance was given to the status attribute most clearly associated with the performance of the group's task" (p. 345).

Although the above studies were conducted outside of personal relationship contexts, one can extrapolate these findings to personal involvements. More specifically, although men prefer a dominant style that they demonstrate through nonverbal behavior, such demonstrations are likely moderated by the task at hand. Those tasks wherein men are perceived as more expert would set the stage for stereotypic male dominance; but tasks wherein women enjoy greater competence or status would likewise present the conditions wherein women would employ a wider range of nonverbal control behaviors.

It is possible that men's and women's use of the same nonverbal message imparts alternative implications for who is seen as powerful. For example, Burgoon and Dillman (1995) examined immediacy behaviors (conversational distance, posture, body orientation, gaze, touch) used by men and women. Men who engaged in the combination of high-immediacy behaviors of close proximity, touch, and eye contact were perceived as more *powerful* than women. When women engaged in the same behaviors, they were perceived as expressing more *equality, similarity,* and *trustworthiness* than did men. Women are effective at displaying dominance at times by violating spatial norms (e.g., touching; Burgoon & Dillman, 1995). On the other hand, Burgoon and Dillman found that women and men can use some of the same behaviors to express dominance. The attributions made about specific dominance behaviors appear to be consistent, regardless of the sex of the communicator, possibly because these nonverbal behaviors possess consensually recognized meanings.

Conversational Maintenance

A widely cited study holds that women are held responsible for keeping the conversation going (Fishman, 1978). More precisely, Fishman reported examples from a conversational analysis showing that women work harder in conversation by talking less, asking more questions about topics of interest to men, engaging in more "back-channels" (e.g., "Oh, yes?" "Umm, humm"), and the like. However, from our point of view, Fishman's image of men is exaggerated, and her use of only three couples (two of which included her graduate students) and 5 hours of recorded messages (from a recorded sample of over 50 hours) appears insufficient to make the following inference: "The active maintenance of a female gender requires women to be available to do what needs to be done in interaction, to do the shitwork and not complain" (p. 404).

DeFrancisco (1990, 1991) adopted the same ideological approach (i.e., a dominance model) as Fishman's. Relying on a conversational analysis of seven couples who were traditional in their gender role definitions, DeFrancisco (1990) reported results that were contrary to Fishman's. Specifically, women (vs. men) talked *more* and asked *fewer* questions, and *neither* sex engaged in back-channels more than the other. Despite the contradictory results, DeFrancisco (1990) reported support for Fishman's assumption that women do the lion's share of the interaction work. Based on interviews as well as the above findings from the seven couples, DeFrancisco (1991) argued that men attempt to silence women during conversation by not actively appearing interested (e.g., showing lack of responsiveness and talking less).

Two other studies (with larger data sets) on the topic have shown that the manner in which men and women maintain their conversations does *not* support the view that women bear the burden of conversational maintenance (Kollack, Blumstein, & Schwartz, 1985; Robey, Canary, & Burggraf, in press). In an examination of roommates engaged in discussions of problems, Kollack et al. (1985) found that male and female roommates engaged in equal amounts of talk (though men tended to speak a bit longer), back-channels, and interruptions. Unlike Fishman, Kollack et al. found that male roommates asked significantly more questions than did their female roommates.

Robey et al. (in press) reported an observational analysis of 19 married couples engaged in small talk about routines of the day or any other topic they wanted to discuss. Contrary to both Fishman's (1978) and DeFrancisco's (1990, 1991) results, Robey et al. found that husbands offered *more* back-channels. In addition, Robey et al. found that wives offered more nonhostile questions and that wives also talked slightly more than did their husbands (though the difference was not statistically significant). Husbands and wives enacted similar amounts of talk time; turn numbers; hostile questions; and confirming, disconfirming, and rejecting interruptions.

The issue of whether women or men engage in more conversational maintenance work remains unresolved. First, it is difficult to compare results from studies relying on different methods. The conversational tasks, for example, are dissimilar. Second, and partly as a function of the need to analyze microscopic indices of conversational maintenance behaviors, sample sizes remain low and prevent strong generalizations. Still, these studies as a group reveal that men—as much as women—do engage in the conversational maintenance behaviors identified by Fishman. In brief, the male dominance hypothesis does not appear to describe adequately the dynamics of conversational maintenance.

Conversational Convergence

Conversational convergence usually occurs when a low-status person adjusts to a higher-status person's language style; for example, by increasing or decreasing speaking rate, pitch, or accent to match the partner (Giles & Coupland, 1991). Reflecting a power differential, the lower-status person is more likely to converge to the higher-status person. Assuming a dominance model, women are thought to converge to men's language style. Mulac and Bradac (1995) suggested, however, that men and women converge to the language used by their opposite-sex partner in a similar fashion. Additionally, convergence on the part of men appears to be greater than convergence on the part of women in close relationships such as marriage—contrary to the power hypothesis (Fitzpatrick & Mulac, 1995).

Mulac and Bradac (1995) examined the power discrepancy hypothesis in problem-solving discussions. They found the hypothesis receives only weak support because men and women did not converge to one another (contradicting results from another empirical study). Men and women's speech styles differ, they concluded, but the transcriptions of interaction showed that men and women have different kinds of perceived power, not dissimilar amounts of power. Women in the study simply did not adjust their language to mirror the men's style. "These findings suggest that in any relationship between women and men, both should be aware that they are using different linguistic styles, but that these styles may be similarity effective in exerting influence" (p. 101).

Sex differences appear to be less pronounced in mixed-sex groups. Aries (1987) noted that the presence of women affects men's behavior in conversational interaction, such that men become less combative and stereotypic; yet, women do not adjust their conversational styles as much to accommodate to men. The male dominance hypothesis, again, seems to be a weak predictor of actual behavior. Differences between men and women, in fact, decrease in more intimate, close relationships. Women become more task oriented and men become more socioemotionally oriented, indicating that partners in established relationships tend to show more flexibility than one would anticipate in their use of communication behaviors, given sex role stereotypes (Aries, 1987, 1996). According to Aries, people's task and socioemotional orientations conveyed through interaction behavior are not possessed exclusively by a single sex.

Interruptions

Interrupting behaviors might indicate one way in which control is demonstrated in conversation, reflecting the polar opposite of convergence. In an influential study of cross-sex dyadic conversations, Zimmerman and West (1975) examined the transcripts of 11 mixed couple conversations and found that almost all of the 48 interruptions were enacted by men. The authors concluded that "men deny equal status to women as conversational partners" (p. 125). Yet, given the authors' orientation and limited sample size, one must wonder whether the clear asymmetry in interruptions has been supported in other studies.

Aries (1996) concluded that "a critical reevaluation of the

literature on interruptions, however, suggests that there may be more studies that report no [sex] differences in interruptions than there are studies that find such differences, and that interruptions may be used for many functions in conversation other than to convey dominance" (p. 80). Similarly, in their in-depth review of research on various kinds of interruptions, James and Clarke (1993) reported that the large majority of the studies found no sex difference in either attempts to interrupt or success at interrupting and that the studies reporting sex differences were evenly split between the sexes. However, James and Clarke did indicate that men (vs. women) are less likely to be interrupted and that women appear to interrupt each other more to maintain their conversations by showing involvement. James and Clarke suggested that the nature of the topic (competitive vs. cooperative) can affect the extent to which dominance-based interruptions occur.

For example, Kollack et al. (1985) examined interruption behavior in same- and cross-sex relationships (i.e., roommates/partners who lived together) as they discussed relational problems (which should provide a fertile context for dominance-based interruptions). Kollack et al. proposed that the *perceived* power balance of the relationship (equal vs. unequal) would predict who interrupted whom, rather than the presumed power imbalance due to sex. The authors found that, in personal cross-sex relationships, men and women in personal relationships interrupted equally. However, in all dyads, the person who was perceived as more powerful attempted and succeeded at interruptions. Additionally, Kollack et al. found that all-male dyads, relative to all-female or cross-sex dyads, produced significantly *fewer* successful interruptions.

Focusing on the manner in which partners communicate control during conversation, Courtright, Millar, and Rogers-Millar (1979) taped married couples discussing four different issues (e.g., events of the day, how to solve problems). The conversations were coded for husband and wife domineeringness and dominance; *domineeringness* refers to one's total attempts to control the other divided by one's total statements, whereas *dominance* refers to one's accepted control bids. Courtright et al. found a moderate correlation between one's domineering behavior and both husbands' ($r = .30$) and wives' ($r = .49$) interruption behaviors (p. 184). In addition, domineeringness for both parties was negatively associated with their self-reported marital satisfaction, although husband dominance was positively associated with marital satisfaction. The authors interpreted this husband dominance–satisfaction link as confirmation for instances of fulfilling gender role expectations.

We must bear in mind that interruptions arise in the exchange of interaction behaviors, and partners tend to reciprocate each other's interaction behavior. In support of the idea that interruptions occur in the exchange of messages, Dindia (1987) observed that occurrences of men's and women's interruptions were highly correlated, and that men and women interrupted each other equally in terms of frequency and kind of interruption. Dindia argued that most research on sex differences in interruptions has not taken into account the interdependence of partner behavior, and that sex differences in interruption cannot be inferred properly until such interdependence is controlled. In short, it appears that in personal relationships men do not necessarily control women through interrupting behavior, despite the common but scientifically unsupported assumption that men in general interrupt more. Rather, men and women interrupt each other and often reciprocate these interruptions in interaction.

RELATIONAL MAINTENANCE BEHAVIORS

Several investigations have examined the extent to which men or women engage in more behaviors that function to maintain a relationship. As with conversational maintenance behaviors reviewed above, one might expect that women (vs. men) expend more energy to maintain their relationships. Two programs of research in particular have examined sex differences. Each is briefly reviewed in turn.

Defining "maintenance behaviors" in terms of how one reacts to relational problems, Rusbult and colleagues (e.g., Rusbult, 1987; Rusbult, Drigotas, & Verette, 1994; Rusbult, Verette, Whitney, Slovik, & Lipkus, 1991) have presented four alternative approaches that they term "accommodation" behaviors. These approaches vary according to their activity and constructiveness. *Exit* constitutes an active and destructive response that includes such behaviors as threatening to leave, actually leaving, and abusing one's partner. *Voice* qualifies as an active and constructive response, and it involves talking about the problem, suggesting solutions, and seeking therapy. *Loyalty* concerns a passive though constructive response wherein the person waits in a hopeful attitude for the problems pass. Finally, *neglect* constitutes a passive and negative response that allows the relationship to deteriorate; neglectful behaviors include avoidance, ignoring the partner, and the like.

In terms of this typology, self-reported main effects for sex differences have been found. As one might expect, women (vs. men) report that they enact more voice and loyalty (Rusbult, 1987). However, in 1991 Rusbult et al. found that men (vs. women) use more voice and loyalty according to self-reports of accommodation behaviors, but that in trained coders' impressions of accommodation behaviors, women were reported as scoring higher in voice and loyalty. Regardless of sex differences, Rusbult et al. found that psychological femininity (as measured on Bem's Sex Role Inventory) but not biological sex predicted the selection of both constructive and destructive accommodation behaviors once commitment to the partner is controlled (i.e., femininity correlated positively with constructive behaviors and negatively with destructive behaviors). Accordingly, it is possible that psychological gender more than sex accounts for one's maintenance efforts, especially when one considers that commitment has a powerful influence on people's reaction to their partners (Rusbult et al., 1991, 1994).

A program of research on proactive relationship maintenance behaviors has not revealed a consistent image of sex differences. Canary and Stafford (1992, 1994; Stafford & Canary, 1991) examined sex differences in the use of five strategies: *positivity,* which refers to acting cheerful, polite, and uncritical of the partner; *openness,* or the extent to which one directly discusses the nature of the relationship; *assurances,* which involve statements of love and commitment; *social networks,* which refers to relying on one's friends and family to provide social activities and support for the couple; and *sharing tasks,* which refers to doing one's fair share of the household chores.

Stafford and Canary (1991) found that perceptions of a partner's maintenance behaviors revealed the opposite of what was predicted based on prevailing stereotypes of women as communal and men as instrumental: men (vs. women) were perceived as engaging in *more* positivity, assurances, and use of social networks to sustain the relationship. Unfortunately, we indicated that these findings could comport with stereotypic expectations, relying on a contrast effect (i.e., men's maintenance behaviors stand out because they are unexpected; Eagly & Steffen, 1984). In Canary and Stafford (1992), however, we found that, when referencing both spouses' responses, wives reported that they enacted more maintenance strategies, and husbands complemented these reports. More precisely, wives self-reported greater use of openness, sharing tasks, and social networks, and husbands perceived that their wives engaged in more openness and sharing tasks. Likewise, when assessing data collected at three points in time, wives self-reported greater use of openness and sharing tasks (Canary & Stafford, 1994).

These latter findings conform to the conventional view of women (vs. men) as expending greater energy in household chores and using disclosure to a greater extent (see also Chapter 3). Yet the variance in maintenance behaviors accounted for by sex differences was typically very small (about 3%). More importantly, equity moderated the effects due to sex: both men and women who felt they were underbenefited engaged in fewer maintenance behaviors than did spouses who felt equitably treated (Canary & Stafford, 1992).

CONCLUSION

How men and women convey control in personal relationships has been examined a variety of ways. In this chapter, we examined the use and perception of power strategies in both influence and conflict contexts. In addition, we examined how control is conveyed in conversational and relational maintenance activities. The literature appears to contradict a stereotypic expectation and presumption of male dominance with regard to the use of power strategies; namely, women appear to invoke a wider range of controlling behaviors, including negative and confrontational behaviors, whereas men appear to act in more avoiding or rational ways. Several explanations for this unexpected finding have been offered.

As indicated earlier, some researchers have interpreted women's negativity as a *positive* relational phenomenon, and that husbands are seen as responsible for responding to wife negativity (e.g., Gottman & Krokoff, 1989; Sayers & Baucom, 1991). This would be consonant with the belief that women are communal and are therefore safeguarding their relationships by using a variety of communication strategies and nonverbal messages.

On the other hand, another group of researchers have argued that *wives* are responsible for withholding negativity: Baucom et al. (1990) argued that the literature indicates that the *wife's* behavior provides the fulcrum for marital happiness or distress. These authors inferred from the literature "two [sex]-related processes": (1) non-distressed wives can and do offer "nonnegative" replies to their husbands' negative messages; and (2) distressed wives "are unwilling and/or unable to provide a positive reply to their partners' negative communication" (pp. 155–156).

We believe that *both* parties are ultimately responsible for each of their interaction behaviors, and that men and women alike can (and should) for the most part choose not to enact negative verbal or nonverbal power tactics and conflict behaviors. Moreover, people's interaction behaviors are highly interdependent, such that the tendency to reciprocate can outweigh the general tendency that might arise from a power imbalance. Accordingly, *both* parties should resist the temptation to reciprocate negative affect and unkind attributions about the partner when they occur.

In addition, we found that—in the realm of close relationships—the evidence regarding use of conversational controlling techniques is inconclusive, partly due to small sample sizes used in this kind of work. The limited data show that women and men appear to engage in similar styles of nonverbal dominance, conversational convergence, conversational maintenance, and interruption behavior. The issue under discussion and the partner's behavior in particular appear to moderate sex differences. People who are more competent than the partner on a topic are also more likely to dominate conversation. However, James and Clarke's (1993) hypothesis that women interrupt each other for relationally promoting reasons should be directly tested and not presumed.

Finally, the research on sex differences in relational maintenance behaviors suggests that men and women enact similar amounts of positivity, assurances, and use of social networks. However, women appear to engage in more direct discussions about the relationship (voice and openness) and they do more household chores to sustain the relationship (a point we discuss in the next chapter). Nevertheless, maintenance behaviors appear to be strongly and directly affected by whether the partner is committed (Rusbult et al., 1994) and whether the partner feels equitably treated (Canary & Stafford, 1992), regardless of one's biological sex.

In short, it appears that sex differences in behaviors that communicate control are affected by contextual issues that moderate any expectations born from a stereotypic understanding of men and women. Perhaps more crucially, this research questions whether men and women are essentially different in their instrumental orientations. Of course, some argue that women are more coercive in personal relationships because they operate from their role as relationship caretaker. Rather than presuming this is the case for all women, and rather than presuming that women respond from a lower-status position to male dominance, we argue that women and men communicate similarly in attempts to control one another—especially in the context of personal relationships.

5

❖

Division of
Household Labor

As mentioned in Chapter 1, several scholars see the division of household labor as a primary location for the emergence of gender-based differences. (By *division of household labor,* we refer to the manner in which men and women assign and accomplish unpaid work in the home.) As the reader might anticipate, the division of labor in the home is tied to historical and sociological shifts in how each of the sexes works outside the home (Coltrane, 1996). The research suggests a recursive link between how the sexes divide labor within the household and how they work outside the home, that is, how work is assigned in the home affects how people work outside the home and vice versa. And as more women seek employment in paid jobs outside the home, traditional divisions of labor appear to be transforming.

Blood and Wolfe's (1960) study of 731 urban couples and 178 farm couples established benchmarks in several aspects of under-standing marriage, including how partners divide housework labor. Blood and Wolfe found that partners help each other to the degree they are available and according to the resources they bring to the family: "Nothing could be more pragmatic and non-ideological than the sheer availability of one partner to do the household tasks. This is precisely what seems to be the prime determinant of the division of labor" (p. 57). Nor did the division of household labor appear to present a problem to married people back in the late 1950s; it was not mentioned among the topics that the participants said caused conflict (pp. 240–251).

Since the 1950s, with the exponential increase of women in paid jobs and careers, researchers have discovered much more disagreement between partners regarding housework (approximately 75% of U.S. women now work in paid jobs). Couples now often report that housework constitutes a salient issue in marital strife (e.g., Gottman, 1979; Zietlow & Sillars, 1988). The issue of doing chores becomes especially "hot" when one considers that present-day women increasingly pursue paid employment and careers, and yet they still are expected to be primarily responsible for performing mundane housework. Feelings of inequity that arise from performing the majority of such work without symbolic or practical support can erode relational satisfaction and individual well-being (e.g., Blair & Johnson, 1992; Pleck, 1985). Pleck succinctly summarized the issue "The family time use problem in two-earner couples which has negative consequences for the wife is not her doing too much, but her husband doing too little. The latter causes the wife to feel dissatisfied with her husband and his level of family performance, which in turn directly diminishes the wife's satisfaction from the family and her well-being more generally" (p. 114).

Enthusiastic but unwarranted opinions about the issue of household division of labor can be easily found in academic books and journals. For example, Manke, Seery, Crouter, and McHale (1994) found no significant difference between single-earner husbands and dual-earner husbands in their housework. However, Manke et al. concluded that these findings "lend support to the notion that, at best, husbands respond only minimally to their wives' employment by increasing their participation in household tasks" (p. 666). The converse of the issue (i.e., wives' concern for husbands as represented in wives' performance of their husbands' chores) was assumed.

In light of other research, however, we must ask whether the picture of husband recalcitrance in the face of increasing wife career obligations accurately depicts most personal relationships. This chapter addresses this question by examining the research regarding the amount and the type of work performed by each partner, the major theoretical views used to interpret the findings, and what current trends indicate for the future. In Chapter 6, we will return to the issue of how couples actively define their gender roles in the division of household labor. The picture one obtains regarding sex differences is more complex than many people might imagine.

Before we begin our review, we should note three problems in operationally defining the division of household labor. First, much of the research focuses on how husbands and wives divide "feminine" chores (i.e., those identified by researchers as stereotypically "women's" work, such as shopping for food, cooking, and cleaning) (e.g., Ross, 1987). The rationale for doing so resides in the findings that such tasks require more time than do traditionally defined "masculine" (e.g., lawn care) or "neutral" (e.g., running errands) tasks. Failing to include masculine and neutral tasks probably decreases estimates of men's actual household work.

Second, researchers often do not count time devoted to child care, nor do they count the help that children offer. Part of the reason for omitting children stems from the finding that children can be both a chore and a pleasure (Spitze, 1988). Because women tend to do more parenting (e.g., Spitze, 1988), not including child care probably decreases estimates of women's actual household work. In addition, not including children's assistance is problematic to the extent that children assume more household chores as they age (Goldscheider & Waite, 1991).

Third, the most commonly used data collection techniques suffer from self-reporting biases. On one hand, surveys of one's household chores for a "typical day" probably also reflect one's assumptions about the "correct" division of labor between the sexes. Moreover, such reports tend to inflate the amount one actually works (Pleck, 1985). On the other hand, diary methods, which typically ask participants to recount their work for the previous week, are subject to memory distortion. Accordingly, we caution the reader that many of the findings are interpreted as if they represent accurate records of actual work when they more directly assess perceptions of work (and thus could be affected by normative expectations tied to sex role stereotypes). Only a few researchers have adopted multimethod approaches in combining observation or interview studies with participants' self-reported data (e.g., Hochschild, 1989).

AMOUNT AND TYPE OF TASKS

Time Spent on Household Labor

Based on her 4-year observation of 50 married couples, Hochschild (1989) calculated that women work an *"extra month of twenty-four hour days a year,"* which when extended for a dozen years represents a full year of 24-hour work days (pp. 3–4; emphasis in original). Pleck's (1985) summary of estimates from the 1960s–1970s regarding employed women's versus employed men's housework verifies Hochschild's calculation. Pleck reported a range of women's overload as 1.3 to 2.4 hours per day, which is roughly equivalent to 28 full days per year. Likewise, South and Spitze (1994) concluded that despite variability in research reports, women on the average perform 70% of total housework even if they are employed outside the home, which translates into about 40 hours per week of housework versus 19 hours for men (p. 332). Ross (1987) found that 76.3% of employed wives do most of the housework, and amazingly, only 1 of 680 husbands she studied reported doing most of the housework. Coltrane and Ishii-Kuntz (1992) reported that men perform less than 20% of the following routine tasks: preparing meals, washing dishes and meal cleanup, shopping, washing and ironing clothes, and cleaning the house.

Although the above figures present clear prima facie evidence establishing that inequity exists in husband–wife division of labor, other information softens the high-contrast view (Shelton, 1990). For example, Pleck (1985) noted that dual-earner husband contributions to housework rose about 10% from 1965 to 1981, to the current 30–35% level commonly cited (vs. 15–20% of husbands in single-earner families). Pleck also reported data from a 1975–1976 national sample; time use (diary) study revealed a difference of only 12 minutes a day (or 3 days per year) that wives worked more than husbands. These data indicate that a precise measure of housework revealed one-tenth the overload of women that has been claimed by other researchers.

Longitudinal data also reveal changes in the division of labor. For example, Maret and Finlay (1984) examined 1974–1976 National Longitudinal Surveys of Work Experience data and found that dual-career women reported significantly less sole responsibility for three chores—grocery shopping, child care, and washing clothes. Using longitudinal data from the United States and Canada with corresponding data from four other countries, Gershuny and Robinson (1988) found a reduction in women's housework of 1–1.5 hours of domestic work per day between the 1960s and the 1980s, *controlling for women's paid employment.* Gershuny and Robinson also found an increase in men's household work between the 1960s and 1980s.

When analyzing both single- and dual-earner families, more similarities than differences emerge in terms of the time devoted to work. For example, South and Spitze (1994) reported that women spend an average of 32.6 hours per week on housework, whereas men spend only 18.1 hours per week on chores. South and Spitze noted that these figures reverse when examining paid employment; that is, men work an average of 32 hours a week in paid jobs, whereas women work an average of about 18 hours a week in paid jobs. According to these figures, men and women appear to be working virtually the same amount of time. Similarly, Ferree (1991) found that both husbands and wives reported that they *and* their partners work about 60 hours per week (with men engaged in longer hours at paid jobs). Ferree concluded, "Because wives do about 10 hours less of paid work and 10 hours more of housework, the overall average difference in workload (exclusive of child care) is trivial" (p. 172). One reason the picture changes when considering all couples is that women in full-time paid jobs do significantly less housework than women who work in the home (e.g., Manke et al., 1994; Pleck, 1985).

Importantly, several of women's chores have been labeled as "inelastic" with regard to when they can be done (Shelton, 1990). Although men and women may work the same number of hours overall, wives' accommodate their daily schedule more than husbands do to unpaid work (Thompson & Walker, 1989). In other words, women (vs. men) more likely pivot their leisure time and paid work around family needs, such as caring for young children, preparing meals, cleaning the dishes, and so forth.

Yet the view that women *uniformly* accommodate themselves to men's schedules overstates sex differences regarding the division of labor. Silver and Goldscheider (1994) contended that women are increasingly turning to flexible jobs that allow them more time to spend on household tasks. Examining data from the National Longitudinal Surveys, these researchers found that household tasks are affected by work-related factors. Women who engaged in shift work and part-time work tend to do more chores around the house. Women who worked in shifts performed 2.5–3 hours more housework a week, while each hour of work outside the home translates into 6–10 fewer minutes spent on household tasks. Age appears to moderate the division of household labor. Younger women's household work decreased as a function of how many weeks they worked in the year, whereas older women's contribution to household labor changed infinitesimally regardless of whether they were engaged in seasonal, temporary, or intermittent work (Silver & Goldscheider, 1994). It appears that older (vs. younger) women are more affected by expectations concerning housework.

Moreover, men appear to be more conscientious parents than some might expect. For example, Crouter, Perry-Jenkins, Huston, and McHale (1987) found that dual-career fathers spent twice the time as did single-career fathers in solo child care (5.3 hours per day vs. 2.1 hours per day). As Gilbert (1993) noted with regard to dual-earner families, "Men's greater involvement [today vs. previously] in relationships, caring, and parenting likely is the hallmark of the 1990s" (p. 43). Examining issues surrounding parental satisfaction, Goetting (1986) indicated that sex differences on the issue of parental satisfaction were inconsistent. Goetting interpreted the research to indicate that mothers experienced more rewards *and* more costs from parenting (e.g., restricted freedom). We should note that child care is not used consistently in the research on the division of labor (South & Spitze, 1994). It is clear, however, that children both contribute to and assist in overall household work.

The age of children in a household probably affects the amount of time men spend in child care duties and the total percentage of chores done by husbands versus wives. By the time children reach 10 years of age, they contribute an average of about 4 hours per week to doing chores, according to one study (White & Brinkerhoff, 1981). Interestingly, from the 1960s to the early 1970s, men with young children increased their child care time; but men with older children in 1975 were doing less child care and more housework than did their cohorts in the 1960s (Coverman & Sheley, 1986).

Research indicates, however, that men participate in child care, especially when they are most needed. Unfortunately, most studies do not examine child care, nor do they distinguish between the two types of family work. As implied above, for instance, Coverman and Sheley (1986) reported that men were engaged predominantly in *either* housework *or* child care. The reasons a man contributes to child care differ from reasons for contributing to housework (Deutsch, Lussier, & Servis, 1993). A father's involvement in child care can best be explained by the mother's work hours and a father's adherence to nontraditional sex roles, whereas a husband's participation in housework can be explained by marital dynamics, such as a wife's marital happiness and a husband's sense of spousal disagreement. Deustch et al. examined pre- and post-natal couples and found that men participated in child care because of necessity, regardless of their own work schedule. Daddy fills in when Mommy's work schedule leaves her unavailable for infant care. This affirms that women are predominantly in charge of infant care (feeding, diaper changing, soothing at night, etc.), unless their schedule limits time spent on child care responsibilities.

Overall, the current research literature suggests the following proposition with regard to the time allocated to housework: Married couples have recently and gradually increased equity in their allocation of housework, although full-time employed women remain underbenefited. Perhaps more importantly, women and men are building alternative models for enacting gender roles. As we show in Chapter 6, "doing gender" with regard to household division of labor involves communicating beliefs and expectations that portray one's gender identity. Before we can discuss this notion more fully, more needs to be said about the kinds of work done at home and explanations of it.

The Burden of Household Tasks

The choice of particular tasks to explore in one's research can affect the findings. On the one hand, one could emphasize tasks that women and men perform separately, which would entail a representation of "feminine" and "masculine" tasks, respectively. On the other hand, one could emphasize those tasks that routinely require the most amount of work but which do not represent any sex-typical behavior. Researchers appear to have moved away from the former strategy to the latter.

Blood and Wolfe (1960) examined the division of labor by

asking participants (who lived in and around Detroit, Michigan) to answer each of the following questions:

1. Who repairs things around the house?
2. Who mows the lawn?
3. Who shovels the sidewalk?
4. Who keeps track of money/bills?
5. Who does grocery shopping?
6. Who gets the husband's breakfast on work days?
7. Who straightens up the living room when company calls?
8. Who does the evening dishes?

Not surprisingly, given this measurement procedure, by emphasizing three masculine and three feminine tasks (with two "neutral") the authors found a relatively equal division of labor. Although item content has changed since the 1950s and 1960s, the presumption of tasks as masculine or feminine still reflects some sex-typical expectations (i.e., that certain tasks, like cooking, are "feminine" and others, like mowing the lawn, are "masculine"). Berk and Shih (1980), for example, found that couples agreed most about the division of labor when they responded to items that reflected stereotypic feminine and masculine tasks, but disagreed most about husband's child care (e.g., husband diapering, disciplining, and dressing). In sum, when couples are presented with lists of tasks that counterbalance sex-related responsibilities differences, then (predictably) the division of labor appears quite equitable.

As Pleck (1985) noted, however, dividing the measures equally between feminine and masculine tasks to assess who does what in the home "highly overrepresents" husbands' work relative to actual time spent working (p. 33). The reason is that feminine tasks require more time. For example, Manke et al. (1994) found that their sample of families spent an average of 2 hours and 40 minutes doing feminine tasks, 51 minutes performing masculine tasks, and 1 hour and 29 minutes doing gender neutral tasks per day. These figures indicate that feminine tasks occupy 53%, masculine tasks occupy 17%, and neutral tasks take 30% of the housework day. Other research indicates a similar pattern: "Women's" work takes more time than "men's."

In addition, and on balance, women's work is quite tedious. In summarizing the research, Thompson and Walker (1989) stressed both positive and negative aspects of women's housework: Women "are unsupervised and rarely criticized, plan and control their own work, and have only their own standards to meet. Women's work is also worrisome, tiresome, menial, repetitive, isolating, unfinished, inescapable, and often unappreciated" (p. 855). In addition, Thompson (1991) challenged the argument that women spend more time in household tasks because such tasks are enjoyable: Housework is not inherently enjoyable; it is typically lonely and boring. For instance, Brook (1993) reported that, among a sample of male and female middle managers in New Zealand, the most disliked activities outside of one's paid job involved routine chores, cooking, gardening, house maintenance, and shopping—all household tasks. Moreover, Brook found that the nonwork disliked activities involving housework rated even lower than disliked work activities, that is, were seen as "less creative, challenging, mentally active, and conducive to self development" (p. 158).

It should be noted, however, that doing housework can have its relational benefits. If tasks are performed jointly, then housework can promote a sense of cooperation and connection; even the most traditional husband occasionally helps with household tasks to support the wife and to offer a sign of affection (Hochschild, 1989). In addition, despite isolation, housework done alone can convey one's love, support, and commitment to the partner (e.g., Ferree, 1991). These positive relational signals of doing housework are also tied to the perceived *responsibility* for who should do the housework (Berk, 1985). If one presumes that housework is women's obligation, men appear to be doing women a "favor."

Several scholars have observed that women typically assume responsibility for housework activities (e.g., Berk, 1985; Spitze, 1988). Spitze (1988) reported findings that *less than one-third* of men *and* women in 1983 thought that women *should* be employed—although a much larger proportion of the women were employed. Directly relevant here, Blair and Johnson (1992) found that 61% of employed wives and 71% of unemployed wives viewed their division of household labor as fair. Pleck (1985) also reported that women normatively do *not* want their husbands to help more. Only 34% of the wives (in the 1975–1976 study) wanted greater husband help, and Pleck could not discover a significant predictor of wives' desire for husbands' help. These findings indicate that women often accept social expectations regarding their gender roles as homemakers. Several reasons explain the acceptance of this responsibility, including the belief that women are more competent at doing household chores (see also Major, 1989).

Perhaps our notions of housework as tedious and dull will need revision. Housework can also be envisioned as *family* work. In this vein, Ahlander and Bahr (1995) imbued housework with a prescriptive, "moral" dimension; individuals in a household, regardless of sex, *should* participate together to keep the household functioning. This approach replaces economic and political attitudes toward family work with a view of it as necessary to support family life. Considering housework as essential to the well-being of a family "may help illuminate its role in reinforcing human identity, establishing viable social networks, and transmitting the definitions, aspirations, standards, and skills that make up human cultures" (p. 66). This statement also implies some variability among subcultures regarding how housework is divided.

Hence, and based on their comparative burden, "feminine" tasks have been emphasized more in recent research (e.g., Ferree, 1991). As mentioned, this emphasis begs the question of who does more, and it underestimates men's housework. For example, Manke et al. (1994) limited their analyses to feminine chores. You may recall it was Manke et al. who claimed that husbands "at best" respond "only minimally" by performing chores. This conclusion is too emphatic to the extent that men's work on masculine and neutral chores—about 47% of the data in Manke et al.—is ignored.

In a similar vein, Blair and Lichter (1991) discounted "masculine tasks" (e.g., car maintenance, mowing the lawn) altogether. These authors offered an index of gender role segregation (*D*) in time devoted to different tasks. Blair and Lichter's *D* is equal to one-half the sum of the absolute differences in time offered to feminine versus masculine chores, with all coefficients indicating the percent that men must change to achieve equality in distribution of all household tasks. Blair and Lichter surveyed couples' responses to feminine and masculine tasks and reported an average *D* of .61, which indicated to them that men (but not women) would have to alter 61% of housework to other chores "before [sex] equality was achieved in the percentage distribution of labor time across all domestic tasks" (p. 99). However, using the absolute value of differences obscures the fact that men performed a majority of several of the tasks that were measured (p. 99). In effect, Blair and Lichter's *D* counts men's work *against* them, to the extent one uses *D* as the percentage of change men must make to reconcile their efforts with women's. Simply summing the differences between men's and women's time devoted to chores would appear to provide a fairer index of inequality.

In sum, "women's work" is often tedious and never finished. Because feminine chores comprise the majority of housework, it is unfair to consider masculine and neutral tasks as equally performed activities (i.e., as involving equal amounts of time). However, to discredit men's housework entirely needlessly exaggerates the data concerning the (in)equitable division of labor. The pattern of men's increasing housework cannot be registered against them if men and women want to achieve equity in the division of household labor.

RACIAL CONSIDERATIONS

Race appears to affect the division of labor in the home. Unfortunately, information regarding this issue in the sex difference literature appears relatively sparse. Nevertheless, what has been written suggests subcultural variation in how men and women divide household chores.

Some scholars believe that African Americans display egalitarian and flexible attitudes toward household work; adherence to rigid traditional gender roles does not characterize the African American family (Beckett & Smith, 1981; Wilson, 1986). In an examination of attitudes toward gender stratification between African Americans and whites, Kane (1992) found that African American men and women (vs. white couples) are more critical of gender-related attitudes and hold a higher level of agreement. Kane concluded that African American men's and women's greater agreement is related to their resistance to racial inequality, exposure to gender inequality, and the degree of interdependence among African Americans. Similarly, Ericksen, Yancey, and Ericksen (1979) examined 1,212 marital couples' division of household tasks, child care, and paid employment and found that African American couples are more likely to share household tasks than are white couples.

For a realistic depiction of household labor in the African

American family, extended families should be considered, especially because African American grandmothers versus white grandmothers are more likely to care for grandchildren (Wilson, 1986). In one study, Wilson, Tolson, Hinton, and Kierman (1990) studied flexibility and child care duties in one- and two-parent African American families and families where a grandmother was present (i.e., was included in the household or lived in the community). Reports given by the members of the 64 households surveyed revealed that even in African American families, mothers complete around 60% of the child care and household tasks. Mothers—versus fathers or grandmothers—reported a greater willingness to use corporal punishment and behavioral management, supporting the assumption that child care primarily remains the responsibility of the mother. Single mothers living alone contributed more work than did mothers of other family types. Interestingly, a father's presence in a household determined how much of a contribution a grandmother made: She performed less when a father resided in the home, but the duties left by the grandmother in these households were assumed by the mother and not the father. Wilson (1986) also supported this finding. He found that grandmothers living with their single daughters were perceived by the household, and they perceived themselves, as active participants in chores.

We cannot conclude with certainty that flexibility characterizes roles in the African American family; studies that focus attention on race do not provide unequivocal support for the notion of equality. African American wives are more still likely than African American husbands to perform most of the housework (Broman, 1988), and white and African American mothers spend similar amounts of time engaged in child care duties (Beckett & Smith, 1981). Nevertheless, comparisons among races help to clarify how divisions of labor may differ. For instance, when compared to white working women, African American working women complete fewer hours of housework (Silver & Goldscheider, 1994). Traditionally, African American wives have worked outside the home and have a higher rate of participation in the labor force than white wives (Beckett & Smith, 1981). African American families have made more progress in adopting flexible roles than have their white counterparts, according to Beckett and Smith (1981). For example, African American husbands share in domestic and child-rearing duties to a greater extent than white husbands, regardless of their employment status; African American husbands spent a median of 5.9 hours per week on household tasks, while white husbands spent a median of 4.5 hours. African American mothers are more likely than white mothers to be employed full time, and African American wives perform only two-thirds of household chores compared with white wives' performance of three-fourths of all household chores.

Division of labor also constitutes a key concern in family life satisfaction for African Americans. Broman (1988) found that those who perform the majority of household work feel less satisfied with family life, be they African American men or any members of the household employed outside the home. Both employed African American men and African American women who complete the majority of the household chores experience less satisfaction with family life. Women, though, were twice as likely to report feeling overworked, and lower levels of satisfaction characterize people who feel overworked.

Other research reveals similar results with respect to the issue of men's versus women's division of household labor. For example, John, Shelton, and Luschen (1995) examined beliefs that divisions of household labor was unfair to women in over 13,000 cohabiting African American, white, and Hispanic couples. Results indicated that, compared to white men, Hispanic and African American men were less likely to think that the division of household labor was unfair to their wives. Perceptions of fairness did not differ among white, Hispanic, and African American women; however, African American and white women were significantly more likely than their husbands to perceive the division of household labor as unfair.

Coltrane (1996) and his assistants (Valdez and Cortez) interviewed 20 Mexican American couples in which both parents were employed at least 20 hours per week in both working class and professional positions and had at least one school-age child. Husbands and wives reported on what they did and what they perceived their partner as doing. Similar to findings by Hochschild (1989), Coltrane and his assistants found that Mexican American wives were responsible for most of the household tasks (i.e., laundry, vacuuming, cleaning, sweeping, dusting, meal preparation, and meal clean up) and child care (i.e., picking up toys, helping children dress and bathe), whereas men helped with the child care and were predominantly responsible for outside work (i.e., taking out the trash, car repairs, home repairs). Coltrane concluded: "To summarize, wives thought they had sole or primary responsibility for many more housework and child care tasks than their husbands gave them credit for and husbands thought they had more responsibility for outside work than their wives gave them credit for. Disagreement was especially likely for frequently performed tasks of short duration that were stereotyped as being women's work or men's work" (pp. 90–91). Coltrane also noted that research on minorities is not necessarily comparable to that of white couples because research on white couples typically reflects middle-class, suburban households whereas research on minorities often focuses on the poor or the working class.

EXPLAINING THE DIVISION OF LABOR

In one of the most comprehensive examinations on the topic, Hiller (1984) identified several explanations that have been offered regarding division of labor. We present six of these as well as related concerns we found in the literature. The reader should realize that these explanations do not necessarily represent polarized viewpoints, as some scholars use more than one explanation in their examinations on the topic. Still, the following explanations do offer different points of view regarding why men and women differ in the division of labor.

Role Differentiation

Hiller (1984) noted that scholars sometimes invoke the proposition that men and women have different capacities for family life, and that these differences in capacities provide a functional argument for why women take on the majority of household responsibilities. As indicated in Chapter 1, stereotypically women are viewed as communal and men as instrumental. Given this differentiation, it would appear "natural" for men to work as breadwinners and women to maintain the family environment. However, as Hiller implied, support for this view has declined on the grounds that clear sex role differentiation has diminished in the United States and that empirical evidence does not bear out such a differentiation for separate innate abilities of men and women.

One example of how obsolete role differentiation has become with regard to the division of labor concerns how egalitarian couples manage the division of labor. For example, Haas (1982) found that egalitarian couples shared a variety of roles, these being breadwinner, domestic, handyman, kinship, child care, and decision-maker roles. Even when egalitarian couples engaged in feminine or masculine tasks in the traditional manner (i.e., without role switching) they "never explained the differences in terms of innate aptitudes by sex or reliance on traditional models" (p. 750). Haas's statement indicates that egalitarian couples see role differentiation in alternative terms; even referring to traditional chores in conventional language does not make sense to them.

Ideological Differences

One of the most prevalent explanations stems from the view that division of labor indicates differences in gender role ideology (Hiller, 1984). Indeed, according to Pleck's (1985) reflection of popular views about the division of labor, a traditional gender role ideology is seen as the "major determinant" of who does what in the home (p. 23). Given that researchers agree that couples are transitioning from traditional to more egalitarian forms (e.g., Fecteau, Jackson, & Dindia, 1994, p. 30), we would hope to see more sharing of household chores in those homes.

Unfortunately, as Pleck (1985) noted, the empirical data do not bear witness to a stable link between one's ideology and one's housework. Although some in-depth qualitative studies have identified egalitarian behaviors (Coltrane, 1989, 1996; Haas, 1992; Hochschild, 1989), the statistical association between one's general ideology and specific actions is very weak (Pleck, 1985; Ross, 1987; Shelton, 1990). Pleck stresses that a liberal ideology does not necessarily reflect beliefs tied to specific housework behaviors. Readers familiar with the "attitude–behavior problem" will immediately recognize that one cannot presume a strong attitude–behavior link without assessing both at the same level of measurement. The same principle applies to the extent that one cannot expect a liberal gender role ideology to predict, for example, instances of planning and cooking dinner on any particular evening.

Power Resources

The third position that Hiller (1984) reviewed concerns one's relative power resources: The person with the greater resources (such as income and social status) can control the division of labor (Blood & Wolfe, 1960). Some research has supported this proposition, though the effects are not particularly robust (Hiller, 1984).

Money might not buy love, but the more money that women earn, the less time they spend on household tasks. For example, Maret and Finely (1984) found that as husband income increases (controlling for wife income), wife housework increases, and as wife income increases (controlling for husband income), wife housework decreases. However, the effect sizes indicate that only 2–3% of the variance is accounted for by income. Nevertheless, the authors concluded that "as men and women approximate equality in the workplace, they will move toward more egalitarian sharing of domestic responsibilities" (p. 362). Coltrane (1996) has argued that this trend has begun. Consistent with this view, young women (vs. their older counterparts) appear to benefit more from resources earned at work. "Young women's own earnings 'buy' them out of housework more than do mature women's earnings, and young women's husbands' earnings increase young women's domestic hours more than the earnings of mature women's husbands" (Silver & Goldscheider, 1994, p. 1117).

Although the speculation that workplace equality transfers to household labor equality may appear warranted, it requires qualification. It presumes that the influence garnered in one domain of behavior merits consideration when predicting influence in a second domain of behavior. More specifically, the resource approach presumes that increases in outside income will consistently register as a positive "credit" at home. Several analyses cite exceptions to the general rule that outside income has relieved women of tasks at home. Thompson and Walker's (1989) review shows that wife income can threaten the husband's self-concept as breadwinner, unless the husband views the wife's income as *supplemental* to that role or as *disconnected* from her "true" role as homemaker. Qualitative data on the topic complement Thompson and Walker's review of quantitative studies to show that sex/gender role identification moderates the effect of wife income on division of labor.

In particular, Hochschild (1989) provided vivid descriptions of couples who enacted variations of traditional, egalitarian, and "transitional" marriages, the latter referring to couples with egalitarian ideologies who attempt to perform traditionally defined sex roles in the division of household labor. One traditional couple, Peter and Nina, experienced tension when she began earning more than he. Both Peter and Nina adopted the view that he had the right to maintain a traditional ideology while she progressed with much success through her organization. Their friends and family were also traditional. Eventually the income Nina earned actually lowered her "credit" with Peter, as Hochschild recounted:

> What was it that had ultimately lowered Nina's credit with Peter and reduced her side in the balance of gratitude? One thing was their joint appreciation of the injury he had suffered to his male pride—an appreciation based on their feeling that a man *should* be able to base his pride on traditional grounds. And this pride hinged on the attitudes of others "out there." Through both their ideas about gender, the outside came inside and lowered Nina's "private account": given what people out there thought, she owed him one. (p. 84)

Finally, Ferree (1991) has argued that because men earn more in their paid jobs, women cannot increase equity by simply working the same number of hours outside the home to obtain the income needed to exchange for reduced hours inside the home. According to this analysis, equality in pay for men and women needs to occur in order for women to use resources as a leverage for negotiating the division of household labor.

Time Availability

The fourth explanation Hiller presented echoes Blood and Wolfe's (1960) belief that the more available partner will step in to do the work at home, given that outside work enables such work at home. As Hiller (1984) noted, this proposition rests on two unstated assumptions: (1) that outside work determines who should work at home, and (2) that work at home is less prestigious. Thus, it might appear to the woman who works at home that her efforts matter less, especially if the husband does not show sincere appreciation.

Regardless of its underlying assumptions, the time availability hypothesis has received mixed support. No doubt, the strongest evidence *against* this proposition is that in dual-earner families men do not "step in" to perform tasks as readily as the availability hypothesis predicts. Most researchers agree that the higher proportion of men's household labor in dual- versus single-earner families is not due to substantial increases for men's, but rather to the drop in women's housework.

One indicator of whether the time availability hypothesis adequately explains the division of labor can be found in residual/leisure time studies. Using a diary self-report measure, Shaw (1985) found that men and women enjoyed roughly equal amounts of leisure time on the weekdays (6.37 vs. 6.02 hours per day for men and women, respectively). During weekends, however, men on the average enjoyed almost 4 hours more leisure time per day (M's = 11.77 vs. 8.10 hours). In addition, one study has indicated that when men work less in paid jobs, they do not "fill in" that time by performing more housework (Coverman & Sheley, 1986). Coverman and Sheley reported that from 1965 to 1975 men's average paid worktime decreased, but that extra time was devoted to leisure activities rather than child care and housework. That is, no significant increase in male child care and housework occurred according to the authors' measures of household labor.

The type of leisure activity presents an important distinction when discussing how division of labor might affect one's free time. Shelton (1992) separated leisure activities into *passive* versus *active* categories. Passive leisure activities are "activities one can do at home as time becomes available. They are less likely to require advance planning or for one to leave the house. Active leisure activities, in contrast, generally require one to leave the house and may require advance planning" (p. 124). Using this distinction, Shelton examined sex differences among the following 10 leisure activities: (1) watching television or listening to the radio, (2) reading, (3) hobbies/games, (4) organizations, (5) relaxing, (6) sports, (7) religion, (8) spectator sports, (9) socializing, and (10) talking (p. 121). Overall, Shelton concluded:

> Men and women have similar amounts of leisure time, and the pattern of change in leisure time from 1975 to 1981 was the same. Despite similarities in their leisure time, men's and women's specific leisure activities vary. Men watch more television and spend more time on sports than do women, whereas women spend more time socializing than men. In addition, especially among women who are

not employed, some leisure time is very closely related to household labor. Non-employed women spend over four hours per week on hobbies, and the single most time consuming hobby is preserving and canning fruits and vegetables. (p. 140)

In addition to the above conclusions, Shelton offered several specific findings that link the division of labor to free time. Table 5.1 presents a sample of these findings.

These data, coupled with the consistent findings that women in dual-earner families work more at home, indicate that the time availability hypothesis applies primarily to egalitarian couples who show a propensity to share household obligations.

New Home Economics

Although Hiller (1984) labeled the fifth approach as "economic efficiency," we prefer the more commonly used title of "New Home

TABLE 5.1. A Sample of Shelton's (1992) Findings Regarding Leisure Activities of Men and Women

Regarding employment status: Employed men have slightly more overall leisure time per week than women. Men spent more time in paid work than women, whereas women spent more time on housework than men. Thus, extra hours at work mean less time for leisure for men and extra hours with housework mean fewer hours of leisure for women.[a] Considering nonworking men and women, Shelton (1992) found that men had significantly more leisure time than women. She concluded that this finding likely reflects differences in household labor.

Regarding marital status: Marital status is strongly related to leisure time for men whereas it is not for women. Specifically, unmarried men have over 4 more hours of leisure time per week than do married men (Shelton, 1992, p. 113). According to Shelton, married men sacrifice leisure time for paid labor.

Regarding number of children: Women with one child have more leisure time than women who are childless or women who have two or more children. Shelton concluded that childless women likely spend more time on paid labor whereas women with two or more children likely have additional household demands.

Regarding age: Leisure time varies with age for both men and women. However, the patterns differ between the sexes. Specifically, men have the least leisure time in their 40s whereas women have the least time for leisure activities in their 30s. According to Shelton, these patterns are associated with paid labor for men and household labor for women. That is, men's paid labor was at a high when men were in their 40s whereas household chores were at a high for women in their 30s.

[a]Shelton's measure of household chores did not include child care.

Economics." This approach underscores how couples allocate labor based on maximization of family resources and productivity. In this view, male and female family members are said to contribute to the total household product according to their individual talents and time. The household thus becomes a "factory" of sorts, wherein individuals should work in areas that maximize the economic welfare of the family (Berk, 1985). Such a goal, of course, can subordinate individual goals to family concerns (Hiller, 1984).

The New Home Economics model presumes that the primary explanation for allocation of tasks is based on the efficiency of family members to produce resources both outside and inside the home. As Berk (1985) demonstrated, homes produce processes as well as products that count as resources. Resources produced in the home include clean clothes, food, and gender identities. More will be said in Chapter 6 regarding how gender is produced through interaction. The point here is that abilities for performing outside work and inside work determine who does what, and gender identities created at home help to institute such expectations.

The development of gender identities at home should be apparent in children's housework. Although White and Brinkerhoff (1981) found that 10 to 14 year-old girls and boys both perform approximately 4 hours of housework per week, sex differences emerged in middle adolescence. Girls (vs. boys) ages 15–17 years did more housework (M's = 6.1 hours vs. 4.2 hours per week). The issue is whether traditional, sex-typical mores are transferred between generations. Research suggests they are.

Daughters learn early to assume responsibility for household chores (Blair, 1992). Berk (1985) noted that mothers transfer their beliefs about housework to daughters. Mothers who subscribed to the idea that they should be "a good homemaker" or that they had "little choice" of doing housework appeared to effect daughters' increased housework (pp. 155–160). Contrary to the assumption that dual-earners directly or indirectly teach their children egalitarian beliefs, Benin and Edwards (1990) found that daughters did *more* work in dual-earner families (M = 10.2 hours per week) than in single-earner families (M = 8.2 hours per week), whereas sons did *less* work in dual-earner families (M = 2.6 hours per week) than single-earner families (M = 7.2 hours per week). In addition, daughters performed stereotypically feminine chores (see also Blair, 1992).

Benin and Edwards concluded that their results "have disturbing implications for each of the family types. With respect to time spent in household chores, *full time dual-earner* families are the most sexist of all family types" (p. 370).

With increases in single-parent families, researchers have begun to address how sons and daughters pick up the slack left in the wake of a missing parent. For example, Hilton and Haldeman (1991) found that, generally, children were much less sex segregated than their parents with respect to household chores. Of the two categories of homes, sons in two-parent homes performed both masculine and feminine roles more than they did in single-parent homes, but daughters in single-parent homes shared roles more than sons did in either type of home, and more than daughters did in two-parent homes. The increased sharing of work roles by daughters implies that they (more than sons) pick up the slack caused by an absent parent.

Institutional Interdependence

The sixth theoretical model reviewed by Hiller (1984) holds that social status in institutions (i.e., labor market, political, educational, etc.) determines who does housework. "Buffers" such as (1) sex segregation on the job and (2) the inability to cross the role boundaries (e.g., between "mom" at home and "manager" at work) disallow much change in the status quo (Hiller, 1984; Pleck, 1977).

One does not have to look far to witness inequality in social institutions. In particular, lower wages for women indicate institutional biases against women holding positions of influence. The lack of institutional status in the labor market theoretically translates into increased obligations at home. In a review of the history of the industrial revolution, Strasser (1980) noted how various technological changes in the 19th and 20th centuries helped to divide sex/gender roles and related division of labor. She concluded, "This is not merely a description of labor in the nineteenth century. Rather, it is a suggestion that during the transition to industrial capitalism, half the population were active participants, while the other half had no clearly defined role in the new order" (p. 46).

Nor have advances in technology lessened the burden of work at home in recent years. Robinson (1980) reported that technology is clearly not an antecedent to the decline in the number of hours devoted to family care by women. Likewise, Gershuny and Robinson (1988) debunk the popular myth that modern machines make life more comfortable at home; instead, "the more technology, the more time spent" (p. 538).

For an example of the second buffer (i.e., the inability of women to cross role boundaries) we return to Hochschild's (1989) couple, Peter and Nina. Nina earned more money than did Peter. In fact, Nina was superior to her peers in a career that required more and more time and responsibility. However, Peter (whose masculine gender identity was wounded by Nina's salary) indirectly required Nina to perform more than her share of parenting. The problem for Nina was that she could not meet simultaneous demands from alternate role expectations. Eventually, following a physical break-down and a plea from her daughter to nurture her like her friends' mothers did, Nina sacrificed her career.

Eclectic Approaches

Researchers sometimes rely on more than one theoretical account to inform their studies. Given that the explanations reviewed above emphasize certain features (e.g., income as reflecting resources and time off as reflecting availability), any multidimensional study of division of labor would appear to necessitate an eclectic approach. For example, Coltrane and Ishii-Kuntz (1992) found that wives' greater resources when combined with less traditional values and greater availability of husbands predicted husbands doing more of the traditionally female chores. Likewise, Ross (1987) found that a wife's employment status, a wife's earnings relative her husband's, and husband education predicted husband performance of household tasks. In addition, husband (but not wife) gender role attitudes were significantly, but weakly, related to his housework. In short, Ross found support for power (i.e., salary differences) and gender role ideology explanations of the division of labor in dual-earner couples.

In addition, theories are sometimes expanded to reflect more of the constructs of interest. For example, Hiller (1984) pointed out that power-enhancing resources in marriage extend beyond one's income. Such factors include social attractiveness, sexual behavior, and the partner's emotional commitment to the relationship. Hiller hypothesized that increases in the partner's affective commitment will associate positively with increases in the partner performing household tasks. Accordingly, wives can increase their husbands' housework performance by decreasing their own commitment and promoting their husbands' commitment. As Hiller explained, "The more independent the partner is, the less likely he or she will be to perform the less prestigious maintenance functions, and the more dependent either partner, the more likely he or she will be to perform those functions. This is the core hypothesis of the power–dependence theory of division of family work" (p. 1011).

In summary, different explanations provide insights into the division of labor at home. In view of the research on each, we believe that predicting household division of labor involves more than one primary generative mechanism or explanation. In some instances, power resources (i.e., wife–husband income) and beliefs (i.e., education and gender role ideology) affect the division of labor. In other situations, resources and beliefs have null effects. Two observations may help explain the discrepancies in outcomes.

First, models for marriage no longer uniformly follow the traditional blueprint. This simple observation has led several researchers to examine family work differences according to alternative couple types. Second, the division of labor in the household appears to be changing, with more and more men accepting responsibility for traditionally "feminine" chores. We now examine each of these issues.

NEGOTIATING COUPLE TYPES AND GENDER IDENTITY

As mentioned in Chapter 1, typal analysis of couples provides a means for understanding the different schemata people hold for their relationships, including gender differences associated with those schemata (e.g., Fitzpatrick, 1988a). Three studies represent how typal analysis can inform our understanding of sex differences in the division of household labor.

One method to demarcate relational types simply assesses social roles women and men have in the household. Relying on 11,016 respondents from a national probability sample South and Spitze (1994) found that on nine tasks married couples and cohabiting couples have the largest discrepancy in self-reported housework; never-married women living at home do fewer household chores than married women (about 17 hours less per week), and never-married women living independently do fewer hours of housework per week than divorced and widowed women. These findings suggest that more conventional gender roles are molded in conjugal relationships, wherein cohabiting couples jointly create gendered expectations (South & Spitze, 1994).

Ferree (1991) used both husband and wife ($N = 382$ dual-earner couples) self-reports of housework to distinguish couples, using Bergmann's (1986) typology. According to Ferree, 38% of the couples were "two-housekeeper" couples, which meant that the husband performed more than 40% of the household chores; 29% of the couples included "drudge wives," who did more than 60% of the housework and had full-time paid jobs; 24% included "semihousewives," who did more than 60% of the housework but who worked less than 30 hours per week in a paid job; and 9% were "cash-paying" couples, who performed less than 20 hours of total housework a week between both partners. However, Ferree also reported that even in egalitarian households the division of labor involved assignments along traditional gender role lines (i.e., women did more of the feminine tasks).

Ferree (1991) also found interesting correlations with gender ideology items. For example, men's (more than women's) egalitarianism was significantly related to how much of the work was shared. In addition, men's ratings of disliking housework were associated with their not doing it, and women's preference for higher standards of household chores was positively linked with women doing more.

Using ethnographic methods over a 4-year period, Hochschild (1989) examined 50 marriages by focusing on how people's expression of ideology matched their routine behaviors. Hochschild emphasized the person's "gender strategy," or "a plan of action through which a person tries to solve problems at hand, given the cultural notions of gender at play" (p. 15). Hochschild reported that gender strategies are comprised of one's gender ideology, emotional responses, and behaviors, the interplay of which between the two partners determines how people enact work at home (p. 192).

Hochschild (1989) discovered three types: *traditional* couples, where the man functions as breadwinner and the wife accepts the primary role as homemaker and does the vast majority of cleaning and cooking; *egalitarian* types, where both partners work on behalf of like-minded values of careers and homelife; and *transitional* couples, where the husband reports an egalitarian ideal but does *less* than traditional or egalitarian husbands to help around the home. Of Hochschild's sample of 50 couples, 10% were both traditional, 32% were both transitional, 18% were both egalitarian, and 40% of the partners disagreed in their gender strategies (p. 282). Interestingly, extensive disagreement between spouses (i.e., around 40%) concerning relational types can also be found in the data reported by Fitzpatrick (1988a). This lack of consensus about the form of the relationship would predict many problems stemming from partners not meeting each other's gender role expectations. Noting that approximately 40% of partners do not agree on the nature of their relationship also implies that such gender-based problems are widespread, at least in the United States.

Overall, these three studies suggest that couple type represents an important discriminator of household division of labor. Ferree (1991) concluded, "Not all wives are adding a second shift when they take on paid employment: some are semihousewives with part-time work who continue to specialize their efforts in homecare; some indeed are drudge wives with the equivalent of two full-time jobs; an apparently growing proportion are in more egalitarian arrangements" (p. 178). Ferree also cautioned that although the optimistic perspective of careers liberating women is naive, the pessimistic perspective that all women do double duty is unfounded. These findings also suggest that gender identities and expectations are differentially recreated.

SIGNS OF INCREASED EQUITY

Structural Social Changes

Coltrane's (1996) analysis of the future of the division of labor indicates that broad social forces appear to promote a more egalitarian division of labor in the home. Although Coltrane noted that "equal sharing of child care and housework is still a rarity" (p. 200), he argued that recent social, demographic, and economic trends necessitate that men do more, particularly in terms of child care. Specifically, changes in attitudes, marriage trends (i.e., marriage timing, divorce, remarriage, fertility, and birth timing), women in the job market, and decreases in outside child care all suggest that men will increasingly contribute their energies to performing household chores. Considering economic, social, and demographic trends and with a focus on fathers in the household, Coltrane offered 10 factors that predict men's involvement in future allocations of family work (see Table 5.2).

Given these broad trends, Coltrane (1996) argued that men and women will continue to lessen their assignment of certain tasks due to traditional sex roles. As a result of more similarity in activities among men and women, Coltrane contended that men's and women's gender attitudes and behaviors will change (p. 224). In addition to the broad trends, men and women currently have at their disposal behaviors and communication strategies of their own that can help define and reify their gender role identities (Chapter 6, this volume).

Investing in the Future

Finally, several researchers have argued, partially in response to children's increased work as they age, that future husbands and wives should learn how to share the division of labor early. Benin and Edwards (1990) concluded, "If parents will start training their teenagers to perform both traditionally male and female tasks, then perhaps the next generation can achieve greater marital equality in household division of labor than is true of the current generation" (p. 371).

One study provides some insight into the reasons that parents offer children for working in the home. In a survey by White and Brinkerhoff (1981), parents offered the following: *developmental* (builds character); *reciprocal obligations* (child should help the family); *extrinsic reasons* (parents need assistance); *task learning* (child should learn how to perform task); and *residual* (various other reasons, such as needs allowance or to keep busy). More than others, extrinsic reasons were reported more frequently than others by parents who were unhappy with their division of labor. Moreover, working mothers, single parents, and those with large families at home were most likely to offer extrinsic reasons for asking children to work. However, social status was associated with use of reciprocal obliga-

TABLE 5.2. Summary of Coltrane's (1996) Predictions Regarding Future Division of Labor

1. "As wives are employed more hours and become more attached to their jobs couples will share more housework and child care." Given the increase of women in the work force and their movement into more professional and managerial careers, women's lack of time for household work and child care is inevitable. Given this, Coltrane argues that men will pitch in and pick up the slack (p. 223).

2. "As wives earn more of the total household income and become defined as coproviders, couples will share more housework." Specifically, the convergence of husbands' and wives' incomes will contribute to a greater sharing of the household chores. Nevertheless, Coltrane notes that only "modest" changes are expected as long as men earn more money (pp. 223–224).

3. "More wives will negotiate for change, delegate responsibility for various chores, and relinquish total control over managing home and children." Again, due to an increase in two-job families, it is essential that men offer more assistance in terms of child care and household tasks. The greatest change is likely regarding men's child care duties, given that women often strive for father involvement for the sake of the children and that men typically are delegated relatively easy child care duties (p. 224).

4. "More husbands and wives will believe in [sex] equality, leading to more sharing of child care and housework." Change of this sort is primarily "unidirectional and uninterrupted." Particularly among young men and women, sex role stereotypes are fading. Still, men's attitudes generally continue to be relatively more stringent than women's regarding sex role equality (p. 224).

5. "As husbands are employed fewer hours and value family involvement over rapid career advancement, couples will share more routine child care and housework." Coltrane reports that men continue to be the primary breadwinners whereas women continue to be secondary providers. However, the notion that men are the predominant providers is losing steam (p. 225).

6. "As fathers become more involved in baby care, they will begin to take more responsibility for routine child care, and a significant minority will move beyond the role of household helper." Although many new fathers will continue to perpetuate a relatively unattached father role, the trend suggests that men are increasingly becoming involved in child rearing. Given that women are working more, men will be expected to (and will) do more. Men's increase in child care will also help to increase men's greater contribution to the household tasks (pp. 225–226).

7. "Couples embedded in loose-knit cosmopolitan social networks will share more household labor. Those in more dense, localistic, kin-centered networks will share less." Coltrane's proposition can be interpreted in terms of economics and worldliness. Specifically, couples who are more cosmopolitan and worldly tend to be professional couples who may relocate often, for professional reasons. Relocation, and other factors (e.g., limited time due to professions), results in geographical and time constraints that contribute to reduced or a loss of time with local kin networks. Employment and college attendance reduce frequent contact with relatives who may have assisted with child care and household chores. Young professionals, for example, often relocate due to career and rely on themselves to complete the household and child care duties (pp. 226–227).

(continued)

TABLE 5.2. *(cont.)*

8. "More parents will delay the transition to parenthood until their late twenties or thirties and will likely share more child care and household labor." This trend is the outcome of changes in attitudes, changes in marriage trends and divorce, the increase of women in the workforce and in professional positions, and the continuance of couples relying on two incomes. Given these factors, couples who delay the births of their children will likely share more chores (p. 227).

9. "High rates of divorce, remarriage, and giving birth in second marriages will encourage the sharing of household labor." Coltrane argues that the once-accepted notion of men being the financial providers and the women taking care of the home and children in exchange is not only changing, but that men's and women's roles are often renegotiated in the event of remarriage. Nevertheless, Coltrane notes that the predominance of women retaining custody of the children will contribute to the woman's increase in chores and downward mobility (p. 227).

10. "Fertility will edge downward and couples with fewer and older children will share more household and child care." Specifically, Coltrane (1996) argues that fewer children likely equates with women having to be out of the labor force for less time. An increase in women working often contributes to men helping out at home. Conversely, women who have many children are often out of the labor force for a significant amount of time. A mother's remaining at home to care for children often contributes to increases in household chores and duties (p. 228).

tions. White and Brinkerhoff concluded that the development of children's values with respect to the division of labor indicates something about the future families of these children as well as the values in operation in their present family. Still, research is needed to assess directly how division of labor associates with values that family members tie to reasons for household work.

Although learning how to perform chores in childhood provides an important way that men and women can learn how to share task roles, it is not the only way. Haas (1982) found that over two-thirds of men in her study had indeed performed "feminine" chores as children. But other men had acquired knowledge of how to do feminine chores in paid jobs (e.g., janitorial work). The lesson here, perhaps obviously, is that learning how to plan for meals, cook, and clean can occur after childhood.

CONCLUSION

Our review of the division of household labor in this chapter is necessarily brief. In addition, many of the research findings may appear quite contradictory. Nevertheless, several in-depth reviews on the topic (Coltrane, 1996; Dellinger, 1995; Gershuny & Robinson, 1988; Gilbert, 1993; Hiller, 1984; Huber & Spitze, 1983; Pleck, 1985; Ross, 1987; Spitze, 1988; Thompson & Walker, 1989), in addition to the studies we reviewed in this chapter, indicate several conclusions and a variety of influences on the division of labor in the home.

At the present, most research finds that women perform a disproportionate amount of housework, although estimates on the amount vary. In addition, and as a result of several factors (e.g., increased status, more resources, less time), women in paid jobs perform significantly less housework than do women who work at home. Dual-earner men sometimes increase their housework efforts, but in most cases the increase is slight. The relative increase in dual-earner (vs. single-earner) men's contribution to housework stems mainly from the fact that women in the dual-earner relationships do less housework than do single-earner women.

Regarding tasks, women perform more of the stereotypically defined "feminine" tasks (such as planning for meals, cooking, and cleaning the kitchen), and men perform more of the stereotypically defined "masculine" tasks (such as mowing the lawn and car repairs). However, feminine tasks require more time per day on the average and appear to be more constraining (i.e., women have less freedom to decide their daily, routine schedule). However, men are more consistent in their child care obligations than with other tasks, though some argue that men's child care involves play as well as work. Regardless, men appear to take more initiative and responsibility for child care, relative to other tasks.

When researchers began to devote attention to the division of labor issue, the Western culture—and specifically the United States—experienced an ideological transition from traditional sex role behaviors to greater egalitarianism. Given this ideological context, the equitable division of labor appears in many respects as a final stronghold of traditionally defined sex roles. Some men (transitional men) who adhere to an egalitarian ideology do little in terms of housework, sometimes even less than their traditional male counterparts (Hochschild, 1989). Nevertheless, other men who adopt an egalitarian ideology do in fact enact behaviors consistent with that ideology by equally sharing in household tasks. Although women and men are both responsible for perpetuating sex and gender role expectations, men (especially white men) generally continue to enjoy a greater sense of power and freedom with regard to household chores. On the other hand, many women do not appear to mind the inequity that many researchers cite and find housework to be a source of pride (see also Major, 1993).

In short, links between social/institutional expectations and individual gender identities are manifested in the division of labor that occurs in the home. For instance, men and women justify their roles as workers in the home often on the basis of their job requirements outside the home, and vice versa. At the same time, however, men's and women's general "time use patterns are converging, albeit slowly" (Spitze, 1988, p. 601). Changes in culture are reflected in the home in a "long-term trend toward increased male participation" in stereotypic female tasks (Pleck, 1985, p. 145). Coltrane's (1996) analysis indicates that momentum is increasing for more equitable arrangements in the future. We think that the equal division of labor in the near future is a realistic possibility, to the extent that people continue to search for alternative gender definitions in lieu of sex stereotypes when negotiating work roles for men and women.

We should mention that scholars are recognizing that indicators of division of labor (such as income and education) reflect rather statically on a dynamic process of constructing gender identities and associated expectations regarding work performance both outside and inside the home. For instance, equity can be restored through alternative communication strategies that vary in their directness (e.g., negotiating responsibilities vs. withholding affection; Hochschild, 1989). Critically, the use of communication behavior to define or redefine one's obligations in the home presents a clear focal point wherein modern gender roles are established, maintained, or changed. For example, the common excuse that one never learned how to cook appears less plausible as an excuse in light of the fact that people can learn how to cook, that cookbooks provide the essential information, and that men may need to learn lest they go hungry. In other words, how couples "negotiate" the division of labor in the home dramatically indicates their gender roles to each other, to their networks, and to their children. We elaborate more completely on this point in the next chapter.

6

❖

Toward an Activity-Based View of Gender

This final chapter attempts to focus on the issues and findings that can help illuminate sex and gender differences and similarities. In attempting to sort through the many issues that have been researched, we reexamined the literature to present an image that supplants the essentialized, stereotypic view that is popular today. At this juncture, we present our emerging perspective on sex and gender differences in personal relationships. Our objective is to provide a process-based view of gender, emphasizing how people construct gender from their daily actions and interactions.

The research reviewed in this book does not support a simple, stereotypic understanding of men and women in personal relationships. The findings instead suggest that differences between women and men in personal relationships are complex and inconsistently documented. Studies using alternative methods and samples contradict previous research; self-reported differences tend to outweigh any actual differences, leading us to conclude that people may perceive sex and gender in ways that are consistent with their existing (stereotypic) beliefs regardless of observed behaviors; and interpretations tend to highlight differences while minimizing similarities.

Thus, the tidy view that men and women come from different social worlds cannot explain the diverse findings reported in Chapters 2–5 regarding men and women in personal relationships.

Still, a few impressions emerge from the review. First, women appear to engage in a wider range of interaction behaviors in personal relationships. For instance, small but consistent effects for sex differences show that *in personal relationships* women (vs. men) are more likely to express a range of emotions, disclose personal history and opinions, use touch to convey intimate feelings in addition to sexual ones, engage in unilateral power strategies, rely on manipulation techniques, and resort to negative and confronting conflict behavior, and they tend to enact the relational maintenance behaviors of openness (voice), loyalty, and task sharing. On this last point, the research also reveals that women tend to engage in more housework and parenting, even in dual-career couples. Of course, these foreground differences remain within the background of many more sex similarities. For example, we noted that much variation exists with regard to the question of sex differences in the division of labor in the home, in terms of estimates that do or do not count men's household chores, child care, racial considerations, and how men and women behave in different relationship types.

Moreover, as we have seen thus far, the research does not support a strong inference that either biological sex or adherence to traditional gender roles provides an insightful or a comprehensive portrayal of findings with regard to sex and gender differences and similarities in personal relationships. Although several theorists attempt to make sense of how stereotypes translate into social roles and interaction (e.g., Eagly, 1987), the findings reviewed in the previous chapters do not support the presumption that stereotypes translate with much momentum into *personal relationship* interaction. Granted, people often perceive strangers and acquaintances through stereotypic lenses. Yet, theorists should attempt to explain the emergence of gender in personal relationships without a reliance on stereotypes and (certainly) without a predisposition toward the dualistic accounts that such stereotypes involve. Research shows that people can eschew traditional gender roles and enjoy more satisfying relationships as a result.

In the following section, we explain gender roles as they emerge through various activities and are implicitly affected by one's genetic code. Our position relies largely on the assumption that people can and do create gender within their daily activities and interactions (for a similar view of relationships, see Duck, 1994). The creation of gender does not ubiquitously follow binary, conventional sex stereotypes. Nor, however, does the creation of gender occur in a societal vacuum. Accordingly, and following our propositions regarding people's creation of various gender identities and gender roles, we present "external" constraints that impinge on people's ability to construct gender in their personal relationships.

GENDER AS CLUSTERS OF ACTIVITIES

As indicated in Chapter 1, gender differences should be separated conceptually from sex differences. As the following pages indicate, "gender" as a social phenomenon can be implicitly affected by one's "sex" (biological status). In addition, gender is a variable process that overlaps at times with one's biological sex. The following propositions outline this view.

Gender Emerges in the Enactment of Activity Clusters

By "activity clusters" we refer to different sets of goal-directed behaviors that people enact. Goal-directed activities vary in amount and types of thought they required (Hacker, 1985), with some goals being concrete and other goals, vague. In addition, activities vary in terms of how social actors perceive their importance and how frequently they occur (Brook, 1993). We should clarify that we do not refer to "activity" as some scholars do to refer to men's "activity-based" orientation to intimacy. Rather we refer to "activity" as an inclusive construct that involves *both* communal and instrumental orientations and behaviors.

Do women and men differ in their activity clusters? Initial evidence suggests they do. Cody, Canary, and Smith (1994) for example, reported three studies that found college women (vs. men) more typically pursue goals that involve charity work, giving advice to parents and peers, escalating and deescalating their romantic involvements, eliciting support from others, sharing activities with peers, persisting when enforcing obligations, and protecting their personal rights. In addition, and consistent with findings reported in Chapter 4, we found that women were more persistent in many of their goals and were more likely to use coercive influence, manipulation of positive feelings, referent power, and rationality when pursuing their goals. Men's activities more likely involved initiating relationships, confronting others about obligations, and interacting with bureaucrats (e.g., traffic officers). Again consistent with Chapter 4 men were more likely to use simple, direct requests as well as avoidance to obtain their goals.[1]

One theory that helps explain how activities link people into gendered groups is focus theory (Feld, 1981; McPhee & Corman, 1995). Feld's (1981) focus theory is "based upon the idea that the relevant aspects of the social environment can be seen as foci around which individuals organize their social relations. A focus is defined as a social, psychological, legal, or physical entity around which joint activities are organized" (p. 1016). Feld argued that foci of activities keep people connected in groups; large foci involve many people, and small foci involve few people.

According to focus theory, the greater the number of compatible foci, the more likely will people become tied to each other (Feld, 1981). In this way, cooking, cleaning, and shuttling children to and from dance class constitute important foci for people, most of whom are female. Thus, foci of cooking and other household chores function as a significant bridge, linking women to other women and indicating appropriate gender role identities. According to the principle of transitivity, when two people independently share a tie with a third party, then the third party will establish a tie with those two people (i.e., "If A and B are tied, and B and C are tied, the triad A, B, and C is transitive if A and C are tied"; p. 1027). Moreover, the likelihood of transitivity increases to the extent that all three people share the same focus. Accordingly, interconnections among group members (within sexes) increase as the result of shared activities.

In addition, once people establish a tie they seek other foci to help maintain their connections (Feld, 1981). In this manner, people pursue new or different activities that become additional foci for establishing gender role identities. Thus, members adopting particular gender role identities seek other foci of activity that indicate they belong in the same group (e.g., Tupperware parties, children's soccer teams, political action groups). Of course, not all activities are similarly constraining and time consuming. Feld argued that constraining, compatible, and personally involving foci lead to denser associations. For example, cooking routinely for the family swallows hours of time and energy, and because women traditionally were given the time to devote to such an activity, therefore this makes it compatible with other types of time-consuming activities, such as attending children's soccer games. Accordingly, routine cooking provides a focus that implicates "dense" group membership (i.e., those things largely done by women). Of course, many women may reject the obligations of routine housework in favor of other foci (e.g., teaching, writing) and would theoretically seek out other compatible foci (e.g., attending conferences) to establish a career-based gender identity. (The attempt to engage in many activities that define different gender roles will likely lead to role strain and, perhaps, burnout; Hochschild, 1989.)

It is possible that men and women engage in similar activities but tend to attach different meanings to them. For example, in Chapter 3 we noted that women more often use sexual intimacy as a means to express emotional intimacy, whereas men more often use sexual intimacy for pleasure. This general trend is certainly moderated in one's experiences in personal relationships (i.e., men also engage in sex as an expression of emotional intimacy, and women also find sex pleasurable). Additionally, we predict that as activity foci merge between the sexes (e.g., as more women engage in competitive sports, and as more men cook and clean), men and women will learn to interpret activities similarly. Regarding the example concerning sexual intimacy, one focus would entail people (friends and couples alike) discussing the meanings attached to sexual intimacy (e.g., that men more than women tend to concentrate on coitus).

At the present, men and women sometimes—but not always—differ in their foci of activities, and they engage in activities that promote the construction of different and varied gender identities. Genders appear to be defined early in life most clearly in the performance of household chores and, secondly, in play (or leisure). In other words, two domains of behavior—division of labor and play—provide two inclusive *activity spheres* that contain foci for developing instrumental and communal orientations, as well as other dimensions that indicate types of gender roles. We use the term *spheres* intentionally to counter the traditional use of the term (i.e., "men's sphere" is defined by paid labor and "women's sphere" is restricted to the home and family).

Division of Labor: The Primary Activity Sphere for Defining Gender

We believe that the primary source for learning and adopting gender role identities occurs in the division of labor. Similarly, Eagly's (1987) "social role" theory argues that the division of labor provides a primary domain wherein gender is created:

> A major assumption of the social-role interpretation of sex differences is that the perception of women as especially communal and men as especially agenic stems from the differing specific roles that women and men occupy in the family and society. The distinctive communal content of the female stereotype is assumed to derive primarily from the domestic role. The distinctive agenic content of the male stereotype is assumed to derive from men's typical occupation roles in the society and economy. (p. 19)

As noted above, this bifurcation of sex role spheres appears to be waning (Coltrane, 1996). Nevertheless, and in a similar manner, Major (1993) noted how the division of labor affects people's beliefs regarding men's and women's entitlements:

> To conclude, I have argued that women and men have differing experiences of entitlement within families, especially with regard to family work. . . . Women's greater sense of responsibility for family tasks and child care reflects and helps to perpetuate social norms and values, and limits women's equal participation in the labor force. Women's unequal participation in the paid labor force, in turn, affects their perceptions of what they are entitled to at home. Thus, rather than being "separate spheres," justice in the workplace and justice in the family are closely connected. (p. 156)

However, we do not contend that alternative foci arising from the division of labor absolutely define men and women in terms of instrumental and communal orientations. Instead, we emphasize that people have several alternative gender roles available to them, and these appear to emerge in the activity spheres of work and play.

The point that gender role identities are largely formed by household chores has been made quite strongly elsewhere (e.g., Berk, 1985; Hochschild, 1989). For example, South and Spitze (1994) concluded their analysis by indicating that their findings are "generally consistent with an emerging perspective that views housework as a systematic enactment of gender relations" (p. 327). In this manner, the performance of household chores offers opportunities to develop foci of activities that define one's gender.

Play and Leisure: A Second Activity Sphere for Defining Gender

A secondary, though critical, area wherein boys and girls—as well as men and women—develop gender roles involves play. Play or leisure time refers to the amount of time remaining in the day after one subtracts the amount of time devoted to paid work, housework, and sleep (Firestone & Shelton, 1988, p. 480).

People's use of leisure time depends in part on the division of household labor. For example, Firestone and Shelton (1988) found that women's *active* leisure time (time spent on pleasurable activities outside the home) was negatively affected (i.e., constrained) by household tasks. Women's *passive* leisure time (i.e., time spent on pleasurable activities inside the home) was less affected by household chores. The authors interpret these findings as indications that women attempt to fit leisure time around their chores at home (e.g., watching television while folding the laundry).

Likewise, perceptions of what might constitute leisure time appear to be affected by the division of household labor. Research indicates that spending time with one's family constitutes a personally important leisure activity (Freysinger, 1994). But for women who assume primary responsibility for household chores, "family time" does not translate readily into leisure time. Shaw (1993) found that women perceived only 47% of family time as leisure, whereas their husbands perceived 74% of family time as leisure. These numbers reflect that wives reported doing more than one activity while engaged in family time (e.g., tidying, cooking) whereas husbands did not report such activities. Even when focusing on time that is totally free of any tasks, wives still reported less leisure time as leisurely (80%), compared to their husbands (98%).

Research on leisure activities of men and women can be traced to the alternative styles of play that adults learned earlier. Vaughter, Sadh, and Vozzola (1994), for instance, found that among a collection of elementary, high school, and college activities, men reported more team sports than did women, indicating that preference for team activities in play extends past adolescence. Similarly, Shelton (1992) found that men (vs. women) focused more on leisure activities involving sports. These findings comport with other research on the largely confirmed hypothesis that sex segregation begins in early childhood.

As Maccoby's (1988, 1990) reviews have shown, boys and girls mostly play within their own sexes, and boys and girls develop alternative rules regarding how one plays and how one influences someone. The segregation of boys and girls into different play groups probably affects that manner in which they respond to each other later in life as men and women in personal relationships (Maccoby, 1990, p. 516). Boys (vs. girls) tend to engage more in rough-and-tumble play, whereas girls (vs. boys) are more cooperative. Maccoby concluded that boys develop relational orientations from play styles that are more *restrictive* (i.e., inhibit the partner, e.g., through boasting), whereas girls develop relational orientations from play styles that are more *enabling* (i.e., facilitate the partner's interaction, e.g., through acknowledgment). In this light, different play styles may account for alternative ways that husbands and wives communicate with each other, explaining interaction problems in marriage (Gottman & Carrere, 1994).

Additionally, research indicates that certain leisure activities promote relational quality over other kinds of leisure activities, and a gender preference may influence one's choice regarding the type of leisure pursued. For instance, Orthner (1975) found that men more likely engaged in "parallel" activities, whereas women engaged in "joint" activities—where *parallel* activities refer to those done together but not engaging each other (e.g., playing pool), and *joint* activities refer to leisure time spent with a focus on the other person (e.g., board games that require discussion). Although not all research reports a significant sex difference in couple leisure time activities (Holman & Jacquart, 1988), studies consistently show that leisure activities excluding one's spouse lead to a substantial decrease in relational satisfaction (Smith, Snyder, Trull, & Monsma, 1988).

Holman and Jacquart found similar results, and they concluded that leisure activities done together with communication are more relationally functional than are parallel or other leisure activities without communication.

We do not naively contend that children (or even adults) choose among play or leisure activities without social constraints. Later in this chapter, we review socially created constraints on people's gender roles. For now, we wish to point out that gender roles are created in activities of work and play, and such activities can often reflect and thereby reify prescribed sex roles (Eagly, 1987). However, again, we view the larger social structures as constraints on, rather than explanations of, the process of gender construction.

Traditional Sex Roles Give Way to Alternative Gender Prototypes

This proposition has provided a major theme for this project, and we now want to examine it in terms of our "activity-based" model of gender. As indicated, traditional sex roles fall along rather polarized, stereotypic lines and unfortunately lead to limited, essentialized understandings of men and women interacting. Such essentialized portraits disallow variation within sexes or within a person (Aries, in press; S. Duck, personal communication, December 1996).

According to the most popular measures of masculine and feminine sex roles (i.e., Bem's Sex Role Inventory [Bem, 1974] and the PAQ [Spence, Helmreich, & Stapp, 1974]), a typical man makes decisions easily, does not give up easily, and is not easily influenced, not excitable in a major crisis, competitive, outspoken, interested in sex, outgoing, intellectual, self-confident, and the like. The typical woman likes children and is relational, emotional, considerate, tactful, gentle, helpful to others, aware of others' feelings, warm, and so forth. These items reflect traditional sex role stereotypes held during the early 1970s; they are due for an overhaul in the late 1990s (Canary & Hause, 1993).

In the 1970s, such scales helped to show that one's sex role identity can emerge independently of one's biological sex, such that a person can be a feminine man or a masculine woman or have high properties of both masculinity and femininity (i.e., androgynous) or neither (i.e., undifferentiated). Still, the concepts that defined masculine and feminine sex roles to begin with were stereotypic and incomplete. The derivation of androgyny as the mix of traditionally masculine or feminine qualities limits our understanding of various gender roles that emerge in various contexts and may actually perpetuate the stereotypes by retaining a focus on stereotyped characteristics of the sexes (Crawford, 1995; Morawski, 1987).

Although most authors believe that gender roles divide according to communal versus agenic stereotypic dimensions (e.g., Eagly, 1987), other research has shown that contemporary gender roles go beyond these dimensions. That is, although communal and instrumental orientations provide initial information about gender roles, people in modern cultures appear to be relying on other dimensions as well. For example, people hold alternative "substereotypes" that represent different types of men and women. Using cluster analyses, Six and Eckles (1991) found several subcategories of the male stereotype: *alternative/no future, philanthropist/gay, intellectual, social climber, career man, lady-killer,* and *egoist.* Six and Eckles reported six subcategories for the female stereotype: *women's libber/intellectual/career woman, nasty, housewife/conformist, society lady, straightforward,* and *vamp.*[2] The authors reported that the male clusters were differentiated by a tough-minded dimension (e.g., playboy vs. philanthropist) and by a reliability dimension (e.g., career man vs. Mr. Casual); the female clusters were differentiated by a progressive dimension (e.g., women's libber vs. housewife) and by a good–bad (sexual) dimension (vamp vs. housework maniac). Noseworthy and Lott (1984) reported similar structural characteristics for women's substereotypes, using a free recall method.

The direct impact of these studies is to show that people use more than the instrumental-versus-communal distinction in their composition of various types of men and women. In our opinion, these analyses also provide indirect evidence that gender roles emerge from activities that are not confined to communal versus agenic dimensions. People also appear to distinguish among types of gender roles in terms of a person's *character,* which is inferred from the person's actions and activities (e.g., reliability, progressiveness).[3]

People hold different gender role prototypes. A *prototype* refers to an abstract model or image that people have for a type of person, situation, or event that is drawn from real-life experiences of specific people, situations, and events (Cantor & Mischel, 1979; Cantor,

Mischel, & Schwartz, 1982). *Gender prototypes* thus represent abstract models that people have for gender roles that are constructed from participation in task and social activities. A couple of distinctions about gender role prototypes are in order.

First, gender prototypes do not reflect mutually exclusive categories. Rather, prototypes represent "fuzzy set" categories, and instances of the prototype vary from ideal examples to more ambiguous examples at the border between categories (Cantor & Mischel, 1977). So, for example, some men can be seen as both "intellectual" and "social climber," whereas other men more prototypically represent "intellectuals" (who do not think about or engage in social-climbing activity) in contrast to "social climbers" (who do not consider or pursue intellectual activity).

Second, gender prototypes interact with sex roles. According to Maccoby (1988), an individual's sex provides a consistent category to help him/her organize his/her gender role identity. However, the gender role identity contributes to boundaries established by the binary distinction of male versus female and concomitant traditional bifurcations (e.g., masculine vs. feminine; instrumental vs. communal). In other words, gender roles are constructed of beliefs, attitudes, and values that are not entirely represented in the language of traditional sex role constructs. In terms of the social construction of gender as a process, one's biological sex appears to affect one's gender role in an implicit manner, a point we develop later.

Finally, one's identification with a prototype involves one's cognitions, emotions, and behaviors (Pervin, 1986). In other words, adoption of a gender role identity requires the person to accept particular beliefs that a "certain type" of man or woman should hold (e.g., the vamp and the lady-killer view members of the opposite sex as prey or pleasurable entities), to respond in ways that are affectively consistent with one's prototype (e.g., the vamp or the lady-killer feels glad when seducing partners, does not feel guilt), and to engage in a pattern of behavior that comports with one's gender prototype (e.g., the vamp or the lady-killer attempts to seduce others and probably succeeds, if only occasionally).

Gender Role Prototypes Reflect in Different Couple Types

This proposition has served as minor theme throughout this book. More specifically, several programs of research investigating different relational phenomena with regard to sex differences indicate that marriage is not a monolithic experience. Rather, people define their romantic involvements a number of different ways, each indicating alternative gender role prototypes. For example, in the area of housework, Ferree (1991) reported four alternative couple types: *two housekeeper,* wherein the husband performed more than 40% of housework; *drudge wives,* wherein women performed more than 60% of the housework while working full time; *semihousewives,* wherein wives did more than 60% of the work but worked less than 30 hours per week in a paid job; and *cash paying,* wherein both partners did housework less than 20 hours per week.

In our view, at least four modern couple types exist. These types approximate Fitzpatrick's (1988a) typology of Traditionals, Independents, Separates, and Mixed (partners with different relational blueprints). Hochschild's (1989) traditional and egalitarian types appear to correspond to Fizpatrick's Traditional and Independent types; Hochschild's "transitional" couple reflects either people literally transitioning from the traditional to the independent form or those couples wherein the wife holds an egaliatarian model while the husband adheres to traditional norms. As mentioned in Chapter 4, Gottman (1994) reported validation of Fitzpatrick's couple types in terms of their conflict management behavior. *Validating couples* look like Traditional couples in their emotional connection and affect in managing conflict. *Volatile couples* resemble Independents in their engagement of each other over many issues. *Conflict minimizers* look like Separates in their emotional distance. Two other dysfunctional couple types mentioned by Gottman resemble Fitzpatrick's Mixed types. Given that Fitzpatrick's (1988a) data suggest that about 40% of her couple types are Mixed, it is possible that other types (e.g., transitionals) can be found by using alternative dimensions to assess shifting gender roles and values.

Studies on martial types indicate that husbands and wives approach each other with very different kinds of expectations depending on the type of marriage they have. That is, one's expectations for self and spouse are largely informed by the schemata that frame the marriage (Fitzpatrick, 1998a). Such schemata also indicate appropriate gender roles. Whereas the Traditional and Separate couples who hold conventional ideologies might not question the presumption that the wife is primarily responsible for the household chores, the Independent couple may negotiate the performance of chores daily. In addition, the use of normative, role-based arguments would probably appear ridiculous to Independent couples (e.g., "A wife should take care of the household, to make sure that it is a happy [and clean] home").

Gender Role Identity Changes over Time

As the previous material has implied, we do not view gender roles as binary products of biological sex—that is, as structural variables that cannot change. Rather, individuals develop several gender identities over time. As Ickes (1993) indicated, one change that appears important to parties in close relationships involves the movement from masculine/feminine stereotypes to more flexible gender roles. Consistent with the view of gender roles as prototypes, Maccoby (1988) noted that

> a gender label functions as a kind of magnet, which attracts new incoming information. Thus, fuzzy sets appear to be organized around core categories, but they do not define the categories. The content of a fuzzy set changes with age and cultural experience, but this does not imply a change in the core category [i.e., gender] with which it is associated. As children grow older, they accumulate knowledge about the kinds of activities they are likely to prefer, the kinds of reactions they are likely to display in a variety of situations, and, perhaps most important, the kind of exceptions there are to the modal trends in sex-linked behavior. (p. 762)

Maccoby's adoption of gender roles as fuzzy sets appears quite remarkable considering that her analysis illustrated many instances wherein young children and even infants prefer same sex peers. Maccoby also noted much overlap between the sexes in their preferred activities and little consistency in same-sex preference over time (i.e., from one day to the next). Accordingly, even when beginning with the notion that the two sexes differ in their preferences for activities, one can envision how both sexes sometimes engage in similar kinds of activities and change the content of their gender role identities.

Maccoby (1988) also distinguished between the binary categories of male and female and the fuzzy set categories of masculine and feminine. For example, playing tennis appears to be a masculine as well as a feminine activity. However, President Theodore Roosevelt refused to have his picture taken while playing tennis for fear that he might be seen in any way as feminine. Instead, Roosevelt posed as a fighter, a wild game hunter, and an explorer because such activities as hunting more likely indicated a culturally recognized masculine identity than did playing tennis. This example also suggests that activities that comprise one's gender role identity change over time—in a historical sense as well as developmentally. That is, as Coltrane (1996) argued, cultures change over time and reflect the shifting activities of men and women. Cultural changes may be clear, though they are often retarded. For example, the research indicates that, at increasing though slow rates, men are engaging in housework and child care, women are obtaining career positions, and women are enrolling to study in men's military academies.

At the individual level, then, one's gender role identity references one's own (focused) activities, which can change over time. However, an individual may not necessarily question his/her sex role identity. In other words, a person can hold one of several gender roles as well as the binary "male–female" distinction (Maccoby, 1988). As indicated previously in this chapter, a comprehensive typology of dimensions that one uses to distinguish among gender roles beyond the masculine–feminine dimension has not yet been examined (see also Note 3, this chapter). In addition, we must consider the role of biological sex in the construction of gender.

Biological Sex Implicitly Influences Gender Roles

In using the term "gender role" versus "sex role" we intend to separate features of one's social identity from features typically associated with one's biology. Yet, being pregnant certainly does affect one's self, is linked to one's identification as a "woman," and excludes men in terms of psychological as well as physical needs that women experience in their sex roles as "mothers." Clearly, biological/genetic differences impact social behavior, though they do not comprehensively explain the dynamics of gender in personal relationships. Accordingly, being a "mother" entails more than selecting a suitable mate, conceiving and bearing children, and caring for children until they are self-sufficient. Being a "mother" for one woman may mean establishing her own (in-home) school to be with her children, whereas for another woman it may mean returning to her paid job as soon as possible to support her children.

In our view, and most of the time, one's biological sex *implicitly* affects one's gender role identity. By "implicitly" we mean that one's genetic code is connected to one's adopted gender prototype without systematic reflection and articulation. Two research examples—the first concerning the communication of intimacy and the second concerning the communication of control—illustrate how an individual's biological sex implicitly affects his/her understanding of gender.

From a social evolutionary perspective, Kenrick and Trost (1997) argued that "initial parental investment" can help explain why women (vs. men) are more concerned about the status of sexual partners: Because a woman invests about 1 year of her life for each pregnancy, she is much more careful to select successful and intelligent suitors, even if she only anticipates a "one-night stand" (Trost & Alberts, in press). But men do not risk such a large initial investment and, accordingly, are less concerned about a particular date's intelligence. Instead, as Andersen (in press) indicates, "Male primates, including humans, are nonmonogamous. . . . Their genetic potential throughout history was maximized by mating with as many fertile females as possible. Though today's males may mate for other reasons than reproduction (e.g., pleasure, intimacy, bonding, etc.), the biology from which contemporary males evolved remains largely intact" (p. 23). More critical to the male than parental investment is parental certainty—the extent to which the male can be sure that the female's offspring are his (Trost & Alberts, in press).

Given these alternative sex-based concerns, some differences have been found between males' versus females' mate selection and courtship (Trost & Alberts, in press). For instance, men seek younger women because men can conceive children longer than women can and men's relative socioeconomic power makes them more attractive over the years. Of course, the evolutionary perspective is only one view—but it suggests that thousands of years of genetic development cannot substantially change in a few enlightened generations (Andersen, in press). Perhaps more critically, genetic differences between men and women appear implicitly to influence how they engage in intimate exchanges.

For a second illustration of how one's sex implicitly determines one's gender role, we turn to research on the physical development of adolescents. Steinberg (1981) and Steinberg and Hill (1978) provided impressive data showing that males increase their power as a function of their physical maturation, independent of their age. For example, Steinberg and Hill reported that male adolescent interruptions of parents were negatively correlated with their age (r = −.29), but the same interruptions *positively* correlated with their physical maturity (r's = .38 for interruptions of fathers and .40 for interruptions of mothers). Moreover, male adolescents' willingness to account for their behavior to parents correlated positively with age (r = .60), but correlated negatively with their physical development (r = −.70). Accordingly, male (but not female) physical development measured independently of age associated with male tendency to stonewall a parent. Interestingly, Steinberg (1981) found that mothers (not fathers) defer to their sons in late puberty, and fathers become more assertive (while sons become more deferential to fathers). Steinberg reported that sons gain in their influence at the expense of their mothers (but not fathers) in family decisions. Similarly, women's smaller physical size provides one explanation for their greater experience and expression of fear, as we mentioned in Chapter 2. Again, these findings indicate that sex can implicitly affect one's gender role identity. The next section stresses explicit behavior that people enact to define their gender.

People Can Create and Recreate Gender Roles through Interaction Behavior

At last we arrive at the point where we discuss research on the day-to-day interaction that helps to create individuals' gender role identities. Given that our model presumes that the division of labor represents a critically important focus of activities, we review the research that explores how gender role identities emerge in the division of household labor. As Thompson and Walker (1989) said, "We will not understand the distribution of domestic work by gender until we know more about the couples' meanings of paid and family work for women and men, and how partners change or maintain the gendered distributions of work through their daily interaction" (p. 857). We agree with other researchers that "gender strategies" present important information regarding partners' ideologies, emotions, and behaviors that define their gender identities (Hochschild, 1989). Such gender strategies convey how communication between partners can create, reinforce, and dissolve gender identities and gender role expectations. The following paragraphs present several interaction strategies found in the literature.

Equity-Restoring Strategies

The literature indicates that women are more adversely affected by the inequity of the division of labor than by the long hours of housework they do (Pleck, 1985). As Thompson (1991) noted, the distribution of justice in close relationships entails examining how that justice is applied. Adams (1965) published several general responses people theoretically could use to restore both actual and perceived equity in close relationships, several of which—not surprisingly—emerge in the division of labor research. Women in particular utilize several strategies to cope with inequity in the division of labor (e.g., Hochschild, 1989, pp. 193–199).

First, women can *decrease their inputs,* which would mean cutting back on work in the home or cutting back on the family. As documented in Chapter 5, women typically do this when they enter paid work. It is clear that many women can reduce their workload at home even more to restore equity. In a related vein, women can wait to bear children, which reduces workload inputs and allows women to garner more income and education and to establish norms of equity before children arrive (Coltrane & Ishii-Kuntz, 1992).

Second, women can *increase their own outcomes* (i.e., rewards). In an in-depth interview study, Dellinger (1994) described how women related that they simply steal time for themselves. As one of the women said, " 'I could find time to do [household tasks] and just have absolutely no time to myself. And I've finally come to the conclusion that I need to do something that is enjoyable for me. Whether it's working out or going for a walk or going out on the boat, it's important that I have down time' " (p. 116).

A third equity-restoring strategy has been to *persuade the partner* to assume more responsibilities around the house. Hochschild

(1989) observed that such persuasion can be either quite direct, as in verbal confrontation (e.g., "Either you help me or we will not have children"), or rather indirect (e.g., by feigning helplessness). Through interviews conducted before and after children were born, Stamp (1994) illustrated how couples use explicit and implicit message strategies to negotiate parental roles. Stamp revealed that the "appropriation" of parenting responsibilities involves messages that facilitate desired actions and messages that inhibit undesired actions.

Fourth, women can *punish the partner.* Hochschild noted instances where wives "punished" their husbands by withholding attention and physical affection. She also noted that women sometimes regretted using such tactics.

In addition to changing their actual inputs and outcomes, women and men *alter their bases for comparison.* To reduce their perceptions of inequity, women often compare themselves to less fortunate women instead of to their partners, noting how well off they are in light of these other women's situations (Thompson, 1991). Likewise, men change the bases of comparison to other men, who "never lend a hand around the house." Conversely, Coltrane (1989) found that egalitarian husbands resisted this norm and instead compared themselves directly to their wives or other homemakers. These studies imply that actual equity relies on keeping the comparison of inputs and outcomes primarily within the relationship.

Research also clearly suggests that women and men *psychologically distort bases of inequity.* For example, Ferree (1991) argued that women's higher desire for quality housework—which was associated with women's increased workload—maintained inequity. In other words, women may value housework more than men do; to restore equity, women may first need to reduce the value they place on housework. Dellinger (1994) called such reframing a strategy of "tolerate and accept." One of her participants illustrated such acceptance: " 'You really have to let go. . . . I think the key is just let go of all of that. If my husband throws his socks on the living room floor and they lay there for four days, then they lay there for four days . . . they're not my socks, right?' " (p. 119). In a similar vein, Coltrane (1989) noted that egalitarian fathers "discounted" the praise that they received for doing what they considered rather ordinary.

On the other hand, Hochschild (1989) noted how couples' rationalized many inequitable behaviors in order to believe that their relationships were equitable. Hochschild described Nancy Holt, a woman who had sacrificed her full-time paid position. Nancy distorted her bases for comparison by cutting back on work (thus she did feel that her "shift" was over when it came time to make dinner and clean the house). She also compromised by using a labeling system that masked the fact that she performed a disproportionate share of the chores—she was responsible for the "upstairs" chores, including cooking and all the cleaning of the house; Evan performed the "downstairs" chores, which only required that he took care of the garage and the dog. In addition, she denied time imbalances, as Hochschild explained: "Another plank in Nancy's maintenance program was to suppress any comparison between her hours of leisure with Evan's. In this effort she had Evan's cooperation, because they both clung hard to the notion that they enjoyed an equal marriage. What they did was deny any connection between this equal marriage and equal access to leisure" (p. 48).

In brief, women and men use strategies to restore actual equity or perceived equity. Energies to restore actual equity and to resist psychological distortion appear to be most effective in achieving an equitable division of labor.

Ideological Biases

One's ideology serves as a value framework for assessing the division of labor. Many couples appear to be quite content with the conventional division of labor, whereas others experience conflict. You will recall that approximately 40% of husbands and wives in Hochschild's (1989) study disagreed about their relationship definition with regard to division of labor. The cause of the disagreement was said to reveal a "broader social tension—between *faster-changing women and slower-changing men*" (p. 205; emphasis in original). Hochschild pointed out that, besides open confrontation, an explicit strategy that egalitarian women use is to verify that the husband indeed holds egalitarian beliefs and acts according to those beliefs. Similarity in ideological beliefs regarding issues connected to the division of labor should provide a framework for shared gender role expectations.

A second strategy related to ideological beliefs concerns how presumed differences may perpetuate unfair responsibility for household burdens. Coltrane (1989) found that equal division of labor was "typically accompanied by an ideology of [sex] *similarity* rather than [sex] differences. . . . (1) Those who believed that men should nurture like women seriously attempted to share all aspects of child care, and (2) the successful practice of sharing child care facilitated the development of beliefs that men could nurture like women" (p. 485). And it appears that one cornerstone belief regarding sex similarities is in place. Specifically, research does not support the assumption that men (vs. women) are more career-centered: Instead, and similar to women, men are typically more concerned with their families than their careers; research indicates that about twice as many men are invested in their families as opposed to their careers (Pleck, 1985).

Outside Support

Hochschild (1989) reported that obtaining outside support was a coping strategy that women in her study used. Such support included reliance on babysitters, relatives, and (for the few) housemaids. But obtaining outside support can apply to moral and social support as well, not only in terms of coping with one's daily tasks but also in defining one's gender role. Haas (1982) found that the social support of friends and family was critical to couples' gender role sharing. In addition, the participants in Haas's study mentioned that their community (Madison, Wisconsin) provided a broad supportive context for role sharing.

On the other hand, many men and women who share gender roles do so covertly, or at least did so in the 1980s. Coltrane (1989) reported that some egalitarian men indicated they feared being seen as uncommitted to their careers. One husband felt he was "in the closet" about the extent of his family work involvement and over 50% of egalitarian couples' *parents* were "confused" about the couples' division of labor. As documented earlier, women have had long-term difficulty balancing expectations of work with expectations to work at home. Haas (1982) found that husbands and wives often conveyed to people that their gender role sharing was temporary ("I'm just helping out with dinner because Janet has been so tired lately") or in other respects not "actual" sharing ("Cooking allows me to eat what I want every now and then"). In brief, it appears that social support is important to couples sharing the division of labor, but that some couples feel compelled to hide such sharing.

Men's Accounts and Resistance Strategies

Of course, men can present reasons why they do not share the housework. Thompson (1991) views such accounts as ways for men to avoid work while maintaining a sense of equity. She provided a list of accounts that men use:

1. Earning wages prevents them from working in the home.
2. They cannot perform the chore as competently.
3. They do not have experience performing the task.
4. They are too tired.
5. They are too squeamish (e.g., to change a diaper).
6. They were not raised to do housework.

Similarly, Hochschild (1989) observed several strategies men used to resist work (though she reported that about 20% of men engaged in full cooperation):

1. *Disqualification* (engaging in distracted and incompetent behavior).
2. *Need reduction* (e.g., "I don't care about having a warm dinner—but if you do, feel free to cook!").
3. *Substitute offerings* (being there in other aspects of the marriage, as in during crises).
4. *Selective encouragement* (complimenting women for how well the house looks and the like).

Despite the above excuses and justifications, research also shows that some men also engage in *affirmation of and assistance with the partner's burden* in the face of stress, which provide a two-fold strategy to increase the partner's outcomes, so as to reduce inequity (Thompson & Walker, 1989, p. 863). As Thompson noted, "What matters to [women], however, is not simply how many tasks they do and how much time it takes to do these tasks. What matters is avoiding tasks they dislike, having 'down time,' and feeling their husbands are responsive and attentive" (p. 186). Benin and Agostinelli (1988) found that men reported that they do desire an equitable arrangement in the division of labor, but women reported that they simply wanted men to help them more with traditionally female chores (regardless of concerns for equitable arrangements for the division of labor).

Hochschild (1989) concluded that women do not push men too much and often give up, to their regret. Clearly, men's accounts and resistance strategies, when effectively enacted, subvert an equal division of labor. The larger, theoretical point is that such resistance strategies explicitly define men's conventional gender role identities in the activity sphere of the division of household labor.

EXTERNAL CONSTRAINTS ON THE ENACTMENT OF GENDER IN PERSONAL RELATIONSHIPS

Our position is that gender is socially constructed and reconstructed through men's and women's activities. However, we are not so naive as to suggest that men and women (and boys and girls) are context-free in their gender role constructions. We must also consider social structural constraints on the activities (and reporting of activities) that men and women engage in to define themselves. Earlier in this chapter, we indicated that one's biological/genetic composition implicitly affects—and in that sense constrains—one's preferred gender role, which we view as a property of the individual. In this section, we turn our attention to the social contexts that appear to us as impacting on the gender roles of men and women in personal relationships. Such "external" boundaries include economic and sociopolitical ones. These are not the only constraints, though they appear to us as the most salient across Western societies.[4] We suggest that structural changes are necessary to provide contexts that foster gender equality.

Smuts (1995), for example, analyzed patriarchy from a feminist perspective in terms of men's motivation to control female sexuality. Although this chapter does not focus on female sexuality, we note that Smuts suggested that people should consider the economic and sociopolitical structures of society in order to bring about changes at more micro levels. Specifically, Smuts suggested that for women to counter men's motivation for sexual control, women must explore political, economic, and legal avenues. She offered counterstrategies for the reduction of gender inequality (e.g., women's political solidarity), more economic opportunities for women, and legal protection of women's property rights. Although our ideology differs from Smuts, we believe that societal constraints affect the creation and adoption of alternative gender roles.

Economic Constraints

As indicated in previous chapters, the traditional division of labor is sometimes explained by one's participation in the labor market. Yet, research is not consistent in its portrayal of men's and women's economic and professional "rise to the top." Some research indicates that women still hit a glass ceiling in terms of their professional advancement (Statham, 1987). Rowe and Snizek (1995), however, argued that gender inequalities in the workplace are minimal. Specifically, Rowe and Snizek examined work value preferences among 4,434 male and 3,002 female full-time employees from various organizations and occupations between 1973 and 1990. They concluded that sex differences are minimal and such "differences" only serve to perpetuate existing stereotypes and myths.

Given the androcentric composition of our culture, however, women still appear constrained by most economic systems (Bem, 1993). Baxter and Kane (1995) suggested that women should reduce their dependence on men in order to bring about more egalitarianism. Yet as Maret and Finlay (1984) argued, women cannot easily reduce their burdens at home by increasing their work outside, because women earn less pay than men do on the average. Similarly, Kane and Sanchez (1994) argued that men's and women's attitudes differ in terms of the workforce and the division of labor at home because equality in the home threatens men's interests. As well, the authors contended that a woman's dependence on a man plays a role in creating interpretations of gender inequality.

Although relational partners often provide support professionally and personally, the creation of gender roles is constrained by economics. Even couples who hold the best of intentions regarding maintenance of gender equality in terms of their personal and professional lives (e.g., supporting each other's careers, education, self-enhancement, etc.), are often overcome by economic need such that it influences or dictates what will occur from a standpoint of "economic efficiency" (i.e., a person's preferences and wants are subordinate to maximizing family economics; Hiller, 1984). Given the remnants of patriarchal hierarchy in terms of power, professional advancement, and wage earnings, women more than men remain economically "one-down." According to Benston (in Malos, 1995): "In arguing that the roots of the secondary status of women are in fact economic, it can be shown that women as a group do indeed have a definite relation to production and that this is different from that of men. The personal and psychological factors then follow from this special relation to production, and a change in the latter will be a necessary (but not sufficient) condition for changing the former" (p. 100).

Specifically, Benston argued that men are responsible for commodity production whereas women are responsible for home and family, an argument often made regarding the stereotypic division of labor. Although Benston acknowledged that women comprise part of the commodity market, she noted that men and women still differ in terms of their structural responsibility; men carry very little responsibility in terms of home and family. The difference between men and women, she argued, lies here: People define women through their activities in the home and within the family whereas people define men through their activities as wage earners and commodity producers. It is within the terms of this structural differential that many men and women define their gender roles, terms that ostensibly limit people's definition of their gender prototypes in personal relationships.

Although conventionalized and dated (e.g., the claim that men have no responsibility in the home runs contrary to other research findings showing increased male responsibility), Benston offered two points relevant to our discussion: (1) Men's and women's respective activities define the genders, and (2) these activities implicate economic constraints on one's gender role definitions. Benston asserted, "In a society in which money determines value, women are in a group outside the money economy" (in Malos, 1995, p. 102). When women join the economy, however, a gap between men's and women's earnings remains (Major, 1989; Shelton, 1992). In our view, this gap will help to perpetuate women's responsibility for the lion's share of the housework and child care (i.e., unpaid work activities).

Assuming the best of intentions between the husband and wife in terms of gender equality, imagine the following: (1) A couple decides to begin a family and must make a choice regarding who will stay home and care for the child; (2) one spouse has the opportunity to relocate professionally; (3) the couple realizes that growth of family and household tasks increases geometrically with each addition to the family; and (4) they decide that someone change from full- to part-time work in order to pick up the slack at home. All things being equal in terms of mutual support for one another's personal and professional needs, economics will probably influence the decisions made. It appears reasonable to assume that the couple will decide that whoever is earning more money should remain working; whoever earns less money will probably leave the workplace to care for the home and children (Farkas, 1976). For instance, the following recent disclosure was offered to one of the authors by a woman who was offered a job opportunity out of state. The woman held an advanced college degree and accepting the job would have been an advancement for her both professionally and financially. Yet, she declined the job offer. She explained: "I would have really liked that job. However, relocating would have meant that my husband would have had to find something new. He's got such a client base built up here, he'd have to essentially start over. It was difficult to pass on the job; but, I have to be realistic. He makes *a lot* more money than I do and always will, even though I'd gone to school longer. I suppose if I made more, things might have been different."

Overall, a woman's earnings must be high enough to impact the family power structure. Huber and Spitze (1983) argued that a wife's current employment status has the least effect on her work attachment, and earnings have the strongest effects on a husband's (but not a wife's) decision making. The authors concluded that husbands may perceive a woman contributing financially as enabling her to have some say in the family decision making. Women, however, may feel that they have a right to decision-making power whether their contribution is through either paid or unpaid work (i.e., housework). Accordingly, one's financial resources affect one's ability to define gender roles, not only to oneself but also to one's partner. For instance, Ross (1987) reported that wives' employment status and greater earnings (relative to husbands') predicted increases in husbands' performance of household chores. However, we also hold that men and women do not define gender roles solely in terms that the economic (resources) explanation predicts, given the low percentage of variance accounted for in the division of household labor in these studies (Chapter 5). Accordingly, economics constrain but do not necessarily explain the emergence of gender roles.

Sociopolitical Constraints

Conventional gender roles hold that "a man supports his family." This notion is embedded in Traditional families as well as the social and political structures. For instance, in 1996, presidential candidate Bob Dole asserted in a debate that one family member "works to support the family," whereas the other works to make ends meet or to pay taxes. This strongly implies that although both men and women work, women do so for supplemental reasons that buck natural law. Even textbooks convey the idea that "dual-earner marriages are often conventional, and the wife's job is seen as secondary to, or less important than, her husband's. Dual-career marriages, where both spouses are equally committed to their jobs and their families, are somewhat rarer" (Pearson, Turner, & Mancillas, 1991, p. 203). Such statements might be mistaken as support for sex role stereotypes that the man *should* support the family and the woman works not out of career aspirations, but out of necessity. Such stereotypes pressure men, such that "manliness" is measured by men's ability to provide support, and it constrains gender choices.

According to Beer (1983), political pressure from both societal and legal standpoints affect a man's role, in that the law also dictates that men must provide support. Beer explained why many men and women often reject the appropriateness of men as househusbands instead of providers:

> Although one of the principal reasons for this is doubtless a belief among men and women that such behavior is not appropriate for men, one of the most powerful reasons is legal. To put it briefly, common law in the United States requires that a man support his

wife and children; in general, married women are not required to support themselves, their children, or their husbands. The fact that many women work outside the home does not alter the fact that while it may be economic necessity or a desire for an income or career that leads women to work outside the home, in the case of married men it is all of those factors plus the law. Married women are not required to support their husbands, and indeed are not required by law to support themselves. Men alone are faced with this burden. In fact, if a man does not work for money, if he stays home and devotes all his efforts to household work, he can be sued for divorce on the grounds of nonsupport. (pp. 93–94)

Women, too, face sociopolitical scrutiny for their choices—choices that are reflected through their activities. Such activities often result in no-win situations. For example, women who opt to stay home with the children rather than work outside the home are often perceived as women without aspirations or goals, or women living off their husband (or perhaps government assistance). Conversely, women who opt for careers without children are sometimes perceived as selfish and too compulsive to raise children. Finally, women who have careers and a family can experience backlash that asserts that being a good parent remains incompatible with activities pursued as a career woman. As mentioned in Chapter 5, the difficulty of crossing the role boundaries (e.g., between "mom" at home and "manager" at work; between an "egalitarian father" and "manager" at work) constrain people from altering their division of labor at home (Pleck, 1977). In this manner, a woman who holds the dual role of working woman and parent is sometimes viewed as being neither a dedicated mom socially nor a dedicated career woman professionally; egalitarian fathers can likewise be seen as not dedicated to their careers (Coltrane, 1989).

CONCLUSION

We have suggested throughout this book that hypothesized sex differences have been emphasized needlessly or because the simplicity of dualistic thinking has been adopted over more complex ways of understanding people and the way they relate to each other. As

Rhode (1990) indicated, "Only by enlarging our theoretical perspectives on difference are we likely to reduce the social disadvantages it has imposed" (p. 2). We concur and take the word "social" to include the manner in which people in personal relationships relate to each other.

As an alternative to dichotomous thinking, we have presented our view of gender as a cluster of activities. Various foci for activities link people who ascribe to one of several gender role prototypes. The prototypes appear to be constructed of dimensional perceptions that go beyond the traditional communal versus agenic dimensions. Moreover, a person's biological sex implicitly affects his/her gender role. We also presented several factors that constrain people's freedom to create gender role identities and gender role expectations.

Nevertheless, most developed nations appear to provide enough fertile soil to permit the growth of various gender prototypes. Empirical as well as critical scholars and social leaders have worked hard to establish the literature base needed to provide evidence for gender role diversity. Dualistic thinking appears obsolete, though dualistic thinking still appears within the frameworks of many people's gender schemata (Bem, 1981). However, the mode of the past is not necessarily the rule of the present, or the future. As cultures develop greater degrees of tolerance and acceptance, people will discard dualistic thinking for beliefs based on alternative models and examinations of one's own gendered actions and activities.

Our last proposition states that people can create their gender role identities through communication behavior. To illustrate this point, we documented how researchers have discovered various "gender strategies" that people use to negotiate the division of labor in the home. Of course, much more needs to be done in other domains of behavior. As Putnam (1982) argued, "We need to design communicative research for the purpose of uncovering theoretical assumptions about the foundations of gender—assumptions that extend beyond biological sex, sex role socialization, and feminist labels" (p. 6). Our hope is to continue to uncover other foci of activities wherein people convey their gender role identities through communication. In this manner, we should be able to indicate more completely a process-based view of gender differences in personal relationships.

Notes

Chapter 1

1. Reis (in press), however, reviewed eight studies that utilized the Rochester Interaction Record (RIR; a diary method for self-reporting interactions and intimacy). According to Reis's analysis, studies using the RIR report a very large sex difference regarding intimacy in same sex friends (d = .85), though sex differences disappear in the RIR studies of cross-sex friendships. (Intimacy was measured with a single item that had participants rate their conversations, from 1 = superficial to 7 = meaningful.)

2. We do not wish to cite researchers who we believe have, for one reason or another, emphasized differences when their data suggest many more similarities or those who did not perform the appropriate statistical test for differences. Later in our reviews of the literature, however, we do examine findings in more detail (though, again, our purpose is not to embarrass anyone).

3. The categories we use here to categorize the existing literature on sex differences related to personal relationships are selective and arbitrary. We wish only to indicate examples of alternative foci and approaches.

4. Of course, many scholars who study the division of labor in the home see the larger society as the primary reason why tasks are assigned the way they are. From an interactionist point of view, the

culture indicates appropriate sex roles for the individual; the perpetuation of traditional sex roles in the home reifies the cultural norms and rules for determining appropriate division of labor.

Chapter 2

1. Although numerous sources provide additional information regarding the various conceptualizations and definitions of emotion, the authors suggest the following as one particularly comprehensive source of information on emotions and emotional displays of men and women: Andersen & Guerrero (in press), and Hall (1984).

2. For additional information on various methods exercised to study emotion, see Brody & Hall (1993).

Chapter 3

1. For a thorough review of various conceptualizations and operationalizations of intimacy, see Prager (1995, pp. 29–42).

Chapter 6

1. Although we do not seek to explain motion (i.e., thoughtless) behavior, we realize that some gendered behaviors could be "mindless." However, we want to understand more precisely intentionally pursued activities that distinguish men and women because such activities can be created by the person in interpersonal contexts.

2. These terms for men were selected to represent clusters reported in Six and Eckles (1991, p. 65). Likewise, terms for women were selected to represent the six clusters reported in Six and Eckles, page 63.

3. Dimensions of work and leisure activities in general—irrespective of gender—include *mental stimulation, involvement of other people, obligation, perceived personal control,* and *stress* (Brook, 1993). In this manner, writing a book and horseback riding are similar activities in that they can be done with another person, are voluntarily performed, and are under one's personal control; yet, these are different in terms of mental stimulation and stress. As another example, cleaning the evening dishes and running on a treadmill

are both relatively boring, lonely, and generally nonstressful. Yet, running appears to be under one's control and is less obligated relative to cleaning the dishes. In terms of mental representations of *gender*, other dimensions noted above appear to complement the general dimensions associated with work and leisure, such as being male/female, reliable, progressive, and good (Noseworthy & Lott, 1984; Six & Eckles, 1991). It would appear that when referencing activities that are salient to gender identities and role expectations, people rely on dimensions that characterize the activity as well as dimensions that characterize the type of man or woman in the activity. At this juncture, however, we cannot speculate about the manner in which such dimensions combine.

4. We acknowledge that other factors partly define these general constraints relevant to gender roles. First, gender roles emerge over time in *history* (e.g., Bem, 1993; Scott, 1996), such that the present sociopolitical structure as it affects definitions of gender is largely determined by a confluence of historical events. In addition, gender roles vary among cultures such that prescriptions for men and women in one culture might be deemphasized in another culture (e.g., Waldron & Di Mare, in press). Also, religion can act as a constraint on one's ideology. For instance, in a Christian manual regarding marriage, the man is advised to assume "headship" of the family (Kippley, 1994). Admittedly, our selection and articulation of these constraints is largely guided by our own focus on how men and women construct gender in their relationships in Western cultures.

References

Abbey, A. (1982). Sex differences in attribution for friendly behavior: Do males misperceive females' friendliness? *Journal of Personality and Social Psychology, 42,* 830–838.

Acitelli, L. K., & Duck, S. (1987). Intimacy as the proverbial elephant. In D. Perlman & S. Duck (Eds.), *Intimate relationships: Development, dynamics, and deterioration* (pp. 297–308). Newbury Park, CA: Sage.

Adams, J. (1965). Inequity in social exchange. In L. Berkowitz (Ed.), *Advances in social psychology* (Vol. 2, pp. 267–299). New York: Academic Press.

Ahlander, N. R., & Bahr, K. S. (1995). Beyond drudgery, power, and equity: Toward an expanded discourse on the moral dimensions of housework in families. *Journal of Marriage and the Family, 57,* 54–68.

Allgeier, E. R., & Royster, B. J. T. (1991). New approaches to dating and sexuality. In E. Grauerholz & M. Koralewski (Eds.), *Sexual coercion* (pp. 133–147). Lexington, MA: Lexington Books.

Altman, I., & Taylor, D. (1973). *Social penetration: The development of interpersonal relationships.* New York: Holt, Rinehart & Winston.

Andersen, P. A. (in press). Researching sex differences within sex similarities: The evolutionary consequences of reproductive differences. In D. J. Canary & K. Dindia (Eds.), *Sex differences in communication.* Mahwah, NJ: Erlbaum.

Andersen, P. A., & Guerrero, L. K. (Eds.). (in press). *Communication and emotion: Theory, research, and applications.* San Diego: Academic Press.

Aries, E. (1987). Gender and communication. In P. Shaver & C. Hendrick (Eds.), *Sex and gender* (pp. 149–176). Newbury Park, CA: Sage.

Aries, E. (1996). *Men and women in interaction: Reconsidering the differences.* New York: Oxford University Press.

Aries, E. (in press). The interaction of men and women. In D. J. Canary & K. Dindia (Eds.), *Sex differences in communication.* Mahwah, NJ: Erlbaum.

Aries, E. J., & Johnson, F. L. (1983). Close friendship in adulthood: Conversational content between same-sex close friends. *Sex Roles, 9,* 1183–1196.

Attridge, M. (1994). Barriers to dissolution of romantic relationships. In D. J. Canary & L. Stafford (Eds.), *Communication and relational maintenance* (pp. 141–164). San Diego: Academic Press.

Aukett, R., Ritchie, J., & Mill, K. (1988). Gender differences in friendship patterns. *Sex Roles, 19*(1–2), 57–66.

Averill, J. R. (1982). *Anger and aggression: An essay in emotion.* New York: Springer-Verlag.

Bailey, W. C., Hendrick, C., & Hendrick, S. S. (1987). Relation of sex and gender role to love, sexual attitudes, and self-esteem. *Sex Roles, 16*(11–12), 637–648.

Baldwin, J. D., & Baldwin, J. I. (1990). Factors affecting AIDS-related sexual risk-taking behavior among college students. *Journal of Sex Research, 25,* 181–196.

Bankston, W. R., Thompson, C. Y., Jenkins, Q. A., & Forsyth, C. J. (1990). The influence of fear of crime, gender, and a Southern culture on carrying firearms for protection. *Sociological Quarterly, 31,* 287–305.

Baucom, D. H., Notarius, C. I., Burnett, C. K., & Haefner, P. (1990). Gender differences and sex-role identity in marriage. In F. D. Fincham & T. N. Bradbury (Eds.), *The psychology of marriage: Basic issues and applications* (pp. 150–171). New York: Guilford Press.

Baxter, J., & Kane, E. W. (1995). Dependence and independence: A cross-national analysis of gender inequality and gender attitudes. *Gender and Society, 9,* 193–215.

Beall, A. E., & Sternberg, R. J. (Eds.). (1993). *The psychology of gender.* New York: Guilford Press.

Beckett, J. O., & Smith, A. D. (1981). Work and family roles: Egalitarian marriage in black and white families. *Social Service Review, 55,* 314–326.

Beer, W. R. (1983). *Househusbands: Men and housework in American families.* New York: Praeger.

Bell, R. R. (1981). *Worlds of friendship.* Beverly Hills, CA: Sage.

Bem, S. L. (1974). The measurement of psychological androgyny. *Journal of Consulting and Clinical Psychology, 42,* 155–162.

Bem, S. L. (1981). Gender schema theory: A cognitive account of sex typing. *Psychological Review, 88,* 354–364.

Bem, S. L. (1993). *The lenses of gender.* New Haven, CT: Yale University Press.

Benin, M. H., & Agostinelli, J. (1988). Husbands' and wives' satisfaction and the division of labor. *Journal of Marriage and the Family, 50,* 349–361.

Benin, M. H., & Edwards, D. A. (1990). Adolescents' chores: The difference between dual- and single-earner families. *Journal of Marriage and the Family, 52,* 361–373.

Berger, C. R. (1994). Power. In M. L. Knapp & G. R. Miller (Eds.), *Handbook of interpersonal communication* (2nd ed., pp. 450–507). Thousand Oaks, CA: Sage.

Bergmann, B. (1986). *The economic emergence of women.* New York: Basic Books.

Berk, S. F. (1985). *The gender factory: The apportionment of work in American households.* New York: Plenum Press.

Berk, S. F., & Shih, A. (1980). Contributions to household labor: Comparing wives' and husbands' reports. In S. F. Berk (Ed.), *Women and household labor* (pp. 191–227). Beverly Hills, CA: Sage.

Berkowitz, L. (1993). Towards a general theory of anger and emotional aggression: Implications of the cognitive-neoassociationistic perspective for the analysis of anger and other emotions. In R. S. Wyer, Jr., & T. K. Srull (Eds.), *Advances in social cognition: Vol. 6. Perspectives on anger and emotion* (pp.1–46). Hillsdale, NJ: Erlbaum.

Berscheid, E., Snyder, M., & Omoto, A. M. (1989). The Relationship Closeness Inventory: Assessing the closeness of interpersonal relationships. *Journal of Personality and Social Psychology, 57,* 792–807.

Blair, S. L. (1992). The sex-typing of children's household labor: Parental influence on daughters' and sons' housework. *Youth and Society, 24,* 178–203.

Blair, S. L., & Johnson, M. P. (1992). Wives' perceptions of the fairness of the division of labor: The intersection of housework and ideology. *Journal of Marriage and the Family, 54,* 570–581.

Blair, S. L., & Lichter, D. T. (1991). Measuring the division of household labor: Gender segregation of housework among American couples. *Journal of Family Issues, 12,* 91–113.

Blier, M. J., & Blier-Wilson, L. A. (1989). Gender differences in self-related emotional expressiveness. *Sex Roles, 7*(3–4), 287–295.

Blood, R. O., & Wolfe, D. M. (1960). *Husbands and wives: The dynamics of married living.* Glencoe, IL: Free Press.

Booth, A., & Hess, E. (1974). Cross-sex friendships. *Journal of Marriage and the Family, 36,* 38–47.

Booth-Butterfield, M., & Booth-Butterfield, S. (1995). The affective orientation to communication: Conceptual and empirical distinctions. *Communication Quarterly, 42*(4), 331–344.

Borisoff, D. (1993). The effect of gender on establishing and maintaining intimate relationships. In L. P. Arliss & D. Borisoff (Eds.), *Women and men communicating* (pp. 14–28). Fort Worth, TX: Harcourt Brace Jovanovich.

Braiker, H. B., & Kelley, H. H. (1979). Conflict in the development of close relationships. In R. L. Burgess & T. L. Huston (Eds.), *Social exchange in developing relationships* (pp. 135–168). New York: Academic Press.

Brigman, B., & Knox, D. (1992). University students' motivations to have intercourse. *College Student Journal, 26*(3), 406–408.

Brody, L. R. (1985). Gender differences in emotional development: A review of theories and research. *Journal of Personality, 53,* 102–149.

Brody, L. R., & Hall, J. A. (1993). Gender and emotion. In M. Lewis & J. M. Haviland (Eds.), *Handbook of emotions* (pp. 447–460). New York: Guilford Press.

Broman, C. L. (1988). Household work and family life satisfaction of blacks. *Journal of Marriage and the Family, 50,* 743–748.

Brook, J. A. (1993). Leisure meanings and comparisons with work. *Leisure Studies, 12,* 149–162.

Buhrke, R. A., & Fuqua, D. R. (1987). Sex differences in same- and cross-sex supportive friendships. *Sex Roles, 17,* 339–352.

Burggraf, C. S., & Sillars, A. L. (1987). A critical examination of sex differences in marital communication. *Communication Monographs, 54,* 276–294.

Burgoon, J. K. (1994). Nonverbal signals. In M. L. Knapp & G. R. Miller (Eds.), *Handbook of interpersonal communication* (pp. 229–285). Thousand Oaks, CA: Sage.

Burgoon, J. K., & Dillman, L. (1995). Gender, immediacy, and nonverbal communication. In P. J. Kalbfleisch & M. J. Cody (Eds.), *Gender, power, and communication in human relationships* (pp. 63–81). Hillsdale, NJ: Erlbaum.

Burgoon, J. K., & Hale, J. (1984). The fundamental topoi of relational communication. *Communication Monographs, 51,* 19–41.

Burke, R., J., Weir, T., & Harrison, D. (1976). Disclosure of problems and tensions experienced by marital partners. *Psychological Reports, 38,* 531–542.

Buss, D. M., Gomes, M., Higgins, D. S., & Lauterbach, K. (1987). Tactics of manipulation. *Journal of Personality and Social Psychology, 52,* 1219–1229.

Caldwell, M. A., & Peplau, L. A. (1982). Sex differences in same-sex friendship. *Sex Roles, 8,* 721–732.

Camarena, P. M., Sarigiani, P. A., & Petersen, A. C. (1990). Gender-specific pathways to intimacy in early adolescence. *Journal of Youth and Adolescence, 19,* 19–32.

Canary, D. J., Cunningham, E. M., & Cody, M. J. (1988). Goal types, gender, and locus of control in managing interpersonal conflict. *Communication Research, 15,* 426–446.

Canary, D. J., & Cupach, W. R. (1988). Relational and episodic characteristics associated with conflict tactics. *Journal of Social and Personal Relationships, 5,* 305–325.

Canary, D. J., Cupach, W. R., & Messman, S. J. (1995). *Relationship conflict: Conflict in parent–child, friendship, and romantic relationships.* Thousand Oaks, CA: Sage.

Canary, D. J., & Dindia, K. (Eds.). (in press). *Sex differences in communication.* Mahwah, NJ: Erlbaum.

Canary, D. J., & Hause, K. S. (1993). Is there any reason to research sex differences in communication? *Communication Quarterly, 41,* 129–144.

Canary, D. J., & Spitzberg, B. H. (1993). Loneliness and media gratifications. *Communication Research, 20,* 800–821.

Canary, D. J., & Stafford, L. (1992). Relational maintenance strategies and equity in marriage. *Communication Monographs, 59,* 239–267.

Canary, D. J., & Stafford, L. (1994). Maintaining relationships through strategic and routine interaction. In D. J. Canary & L. Stafford (Eds.), *Communication and relational maintenance* (pp. 3–22). San Diego: Academic Press.

Cantor, N., & Mischel, W. (1977). Traits as prototypes: Effects on recognition memory. *Journal of Personality and Social Psychology, 35,* 38–48.

Cantor, N., & Mischel, W. (1979). Prototypes in person perception. In L. Berkowitz (Ed.), *Advances in experimental social psychology* (Vol. 12, pp. 3–52). New York: Academic Press.

Cantor, N., Mischel, W., & Schwartz, J. (1982). A prototype analysis of situations. *Cognitive psychology, 14,* 45–77.

Chambless, D. L. (1982). Characteristics of agoraphobics. In D. L. Chambless & A. J. Goldstein (Eds.), *Agoraphobia: Multiple perspectives on theory and treatment.* New York: Wiley.

Christensen, A., & Heavey, C. L. (1990). Gender and social structure in the demand/withdrawal pattern of marital conflict. *Journal of Personality and Social Psychology, 59,* 73–81.

Clark, R. D. (1990). The impact of AIDS on gender differences in willingness to engage in casual sex. *Journal of Applied Social Psychology, 20,* 771–782.

Cody, M. J., Canary, D. J., & Smith, S. (1994). Compliance-gaining goals: An inductive analysis of actors' goal types, strategies, and successes. In J. A. Daly & J. M. Wiemann (Eds.), *Strategic interpersonal communication.* Hillsdale, NJ: Erlbaum.

Coltrane, S. (1989). Household labor and the routine production of gender. *Social Problems, 36,* 473–490.

Coltrane, S. (1996). *Family man.* New York: Oxford University Press.

Coltrane, S., & Ishii-Kuntz, M. (1992). Men's housework: A life course perspective. *Journal of Marriage and the Family, 54,* 43–57.

Conway, M., Giannopoulos, C., Stiefenhofer, K. (1990). Response styles to sadness are related to sex and sex-role orientation. *Sex Roles, 22*(9–10), 579–587.

Cooney, T. M., & Uhlenberg, P. (1991). Changes in work–family connections among highly educated men and women. *Journal of Family Issues, 12,* 69–90.

Courtright, J. A., Millar, F. E., & Rogers-Millar, L. E. (1979). Domineeringness and dominance: Replication and expansion. *Communication Monographs, 46,* 179–192.

Coverman, S., & Sheley, J. F. (1986). Change in men's housework and child-care time, 1965–1975. *Journal of Marriage and the Family, 48,* 413–422.

Crawford, M. (1995). *Talking difference: On gender and language.* Thousand Oaks, CA: Sage.

Critelli, J. W., Myers, E. J., & Loos, V. E. (1986). The components of love: Romantic attraction and sex role orientation. *Journal of Personality, 54,* 354–370.

Crouter, A., Perry-Jenkins, M., Huston, T., & McHale, S. (1987). Processes underlying father involvement in dual-earner and single-earner families. *Developmental Psychology, 23,* 431–440.

Cupach, W. R., & Canary, D. J. (1995). Managing conflict and anger: Investigating the sex stereotype hypothesis. In P. J. Kalbfleisch & M. J.

Cody (Eds.), *Gender, power, and communication in human relationships* (pp. 233–252). Hillsdale, NJ: Erlbaum.

Davis, M. S. (1973). *Intimate relations.* New York: Free Press.

DeFrancisco, V. L. (1990, November). *Response to Pamela Fishman: A qualitative study of on-going interactions in heterosexual couples' homes.* Paper presented at the Speech Communication Association Convention, Chicago, IL.

DeFrancisco, V. L. (1991). The sounds of silence: How men silence women in marital relations. *Discourse and Society, 2,* 413–423.

Deaux, K. (1984). From individual differences to social categories: Analysis of a decade's research on gender. *American Psychologist, 39,* 105–116.

Deaux, K. (1985). Sex and gender. *Annual Review of Psychology, 36,* 49–81.

Deaux, K., & Lewis, L. L. (1984). The structure of gender stereotypes: Interrelationships among components and gender label. *Journal of Personality and Social Psychology, 46,* 991–1004.

Deaux, K., & Major, B. (1987). Putting gender into context: An interactive model of gender-related behavior. *Psychological Review, 94,* 369–389.

Deaux, K., & Major, B. (1990). A social-psychological model of gender. In D. L. Rhode (Ed.), *Theoretical perspectives on sexual difference* (pp. 89–99). New Haven, CT: Yale University Press.

Dellinger, C. (1994). *How women make sense of household task allocation: An inductive analysis.* Unpublished doctoral dissertation, Ohio University, Athens, OH.

Delp, M., & Sackheim, H. A. (1987). Effects of mood on lacrimal flow: Sex differences and asymmetry. *Psychophysiology, 24*(5), 550–556.

de Rivera, J., & Grinkis, C. (1986). Emotions as social relationships. *Motivation and Emotion, 10*(4), 351–369.

Derlega, V. J., Durham, B., Gockel, B., & Sholis, D. (1981). Sex differences in self-disclosure: Effects of topic content, friendship, and partner's sex. *Sex Roles, 7,* 433–447.

Deutsch, F. M., Lussier, J. B., & Servis, L. J. (1993). Husbands at home: Predictors of paternal participation in child care and housework. *Journal of Personality and Social Psychology, 65,* 1154–1166.

Dillon, K. M., Wolf, E., & Katz, H. (1985). Sex roles, gender, and fear. *Journal of Psychology, 119*(4), 355–359.

Dindia, K. (1987). The effects of sex of subject and sex of partner on interruptions. *Human Communication Research, 13,* 345-371.

Dindia, K. (1994). A multiphasic view of relationship maintenance strategies. In D. J. Canary & L. Stafford (Eds.), *Communication and relational maintenance* (pp. 91–112). San Diego: Academic Press.

Dindia, K., & Allen, M. (1992). Sex differences in self-disclosure: A meta-analysis. *Psychological Bulletin, 112,* 106–124.

Dion, K. K., & Dion, K. L. (1993). Individualistic and collectivistic perspectives on gender and the cultural context of love and intimacy. *Journal of Social Issues, 49*(3), 53–69.

Dore', F. Y., & Kirouac, G. (1985). Identifying the eliciting situations of six fundamental emotions. *Journal of Psychology, 119*(5), 423–440.

Dosser, D., Balswick, J., & Halverson, C. (1986). Male inexpressiveness and relationships. *Journal of Social and Personal Relationships, 3,* 241–256.

Dovido, J. F., Ellyson, S. L., Keating, C. F., Heltman, K., & Brown, C. E. (1988). The relationship of social power to visual displays of dominance between men and women. *Journal of Personality and Social Psychology, 54,* 233–242.

Duck, S. W. (1990). Relationships as unfinished business: Out of the frying pan and into the 1990s. *Journal of Social and Personal Relationships, 7,* 5–24.

Duck, S. W. (1991). *Understanding relationships.* New York: Guilford Press.

Duck, S. (1994). *Meaningful relationships: Talking, sense, and relating.* Thousand Oaks, CA: Sage.

Duck, S., Rutt, D. J., Hurst, M., & Strejc, H. (1991). Some evident truths about communication in everyday relationships: All communication is not created equal. *Human Communication Research, 18,* 228–267.

Duck, S., & Wright, P. (1993). Reexamining gender differences in same-gender friendships: A close look at two kinds of data. *Sex Roles, 28,* 709–727.

Eagly, A. H. (1987). *Sex differences in social behavior: A social-role interpretation.* Hillsdale, NJ: Erlbaum.

Eagly, A. H. (1995). The science and politics of comparing women and men. *American Psychologist, 50,* 145–158.

Eagly, A. H., & Carli, L. L. (1981). Sex of researchers and sex-typed communications as determinants of sex differences in influenceability: A meta-analysis. *Psychological Bulletin, 90,* 1–20.

Eagly, A. H., & Crowley, M. (1986). Gender and helping behavior: A meta-analytic review of the social psychological literature. *Psychological Bulletin, 100,* 283–308.

Eagly, A. H., & Johnson, B. T. (1990). Gender and leadership style: A meta-analysis. *Psychological Bulletin, 108,* 233–256.

Eagly, A. H., & Karau, S. J. (1991). Gender and the emergence of leaders: A meta-analysis. *Journal of Personality and Social Psychology, 60,* 685–710.

Eagly, A. H., Makhijani, M. G., & Klonsky, B. G. (1992). Gender and evaluation of leaders: A meta-analysis. *Psychological Bulletin, 111,* 3–22.

Eagly, A. H., & Steffen, V. (1984). Gender stereotypes stem from the distribution of women and men into social roles. *Journal of Personality and Social Psychology, 46,* 735–754.

Eagly, A. H., & Steffen, V. (1986). Gender and aggressive behavior: A meta-analytic review of the social psychological literature. *Psychological Bulletin, 100,* 309–330.

Egerton, M. (1988). Passionate women and passionate men: Sex differences in accounting for angry and weeping episodes. *British Journal of Social Psychology, 27,* 51–66.

Eisler, R. M., Skidmore, J. R., & Ward, C. H. (1988). Masculine gender-role stress: Predictor of anger, anxiety, and health-risk behaviors. *Journal of Personality Assessment, 52*(1), 133–141.

Ekman, P., & Friesen, W. V. (1978). *The facial action coding system.* Palo Alto, CA: Consulting Psychologists Press.

Ekman, P., & Friesen, W. V. (1982). Felt, false, and miserable smiles. *Journal of Nonverbal Behavior, 6*(4), 238–252.

Ekman, P., & Friesen, W. V. (1986). A new pan-cultural facial expression of emotion. *Motivation and Emotion, 10,* 159–168.

Ekman, P., Friesen, W. V., & O'Sullivan, M. (1988). Smiles when lying. *Journal of Personality and Social Psychology, 54,* 414–420.

Ekman, P., Levenson, R. W., & Friesen, W. V. (1983). Autonomic nervous system activity distinguishes among emotions. *Science, 221,* 1208–1210.

Emmers, T. M., & Dindia, K. (1995). The effect of relational stage and intimacy on touch: An extension of Guerrero and Andersen. *Personal Relationships, 2,* 225–236.

Emmons, R. A., & Diener, E. (1986). An interactional approach to the study of personality and emotion. *Journal of Personality, 54*(2), 371–384.

Ericksen, J. A., Yancey, W. L., & Ericksen, E. P. (1979). The division of family roles. *Journal of Marriage and the Family, 41,* 301–311.

Exline, R. V. (1963). Explorations in the process of personal perception: Visual interaction in relation to competition, sex, and need for affiliation. *Journal of Personality, 31,* 1–20.

Falbo, T., & Peplau, L. A. (1980). Power strategies in intimate relationships. *Journal of Personality and Social Psychology, 38,* 618–628.

Farkas, G. (1976). Education, wage rates, and the division of labor between husband and wife. *Journal of Marriage and the Family, 38,* 473–483.

Fecteau, T. J., Jackson, J., & Dindia, K. (1994). Gender orientation scales: An empirical assessment of content validity. In L. A. M. Perry, L. H. Turner, & H. M. Sterk (Eds.), *Constructing and reconstructing gender: The links among career, language, and gender* (pp. 17–34). Albany: State University of New York Press.

Fehr, B. (1993). How do I love thee? Let me consult my prototype. In S. Duck (Ed.), *Individuals in relationships* (pp. 87–120). Newbury Park, CA: Sage.

Fehr, B. (1996). *Friendship processes.* Thousand Oaks, CA: Sage.

Fehr, B., & Russell, J. A. (1984). Concept of emotion viewed from a prototype perspective. *Journal of Experimental Psychology: General, 113,* 464–486.

Feld, S. (1981). The focussed organization of social ties. *American Journal of Sociology, 86,* 1015–1035.

Felmlee, D. H. (1994). Who's on top? Power in romantic relationships. *Sex Roles, 31,* 275–295.

Ferree, M. M. (1991). The gender division of labor in two-earner marriages: Dimensions of variability and change. *Journal of Family Issues, 12,* 158–180.

Firestone, J., & Shelton, B. A. (1988). An estimation of the effects of women's work on available leisure time. *Journal of Family Issues, 9,* 478–495.

Fisher, B. A. (1983). Differential effects of sexual composition and interactional context on interaction patterns in dyads. *Human Communication Research, 9,* 225–238.

Fishman, P. (1978). Interaction: The work women do. *Social Problems, 25,* 397–406.

Fitzpatrick, M. A. (1988a). *Between husbands and wives: Communication in marriage.* Newbury Park, CA: Sage.

Fitzpatrick, M. A. (1988b). Negotiation, problem solving and conflict in various types of marriages. In P. Noller & M. A. Fitzpatrick (Eds.), *Perspectives on marital interaction* (pp. 245–270). Philadelphia: Multilingual Matters.

Fitzpatrick, M. A., & Mulac, A. (1995). Relating to spouse and stranger: Gender-preferential language use. In P. J. Kalbfleisch & M. J. Cody (Eds.), *Gender, power, and communication in human relationships* (pp. 213–231). Hillsdale, NJ: Erlbaum.

Fitzpatrick, M. A., & Winke, T. (1979). You always hurt the one you love: Strategies and tactics in interpersonal conflict. *Communication Quarterly, 27,* 3–11.

Foa, U. G., Anderson, B., Converse, J., Urbansky, W. A., Cawley, M. J., Muhlhausen, S. M., & Tornblom, K. Y. (1987). Gender-related sexual attitudes: Some cross-cultural similarities and differences. *Sex Roles, 16*(9–10), 511–519.

Freysinger, V. J. (1994). Leisure with children and parental satisfaction: Further evidence of a sex difference in the experience of adult roles and leisure. *Journal of Leisure Research, 26,* 212–226.

Friedman, H. S., & Miller-Herringer, T. (1991). Nonverbal display of emotion in public and private: Self-monitoring, personality, and expressive cues. *Journal of Personality and Social Psychology, 1*(5), 766–775.

Frijda, N. H., Kuipers, P., & ter Shure, E. (1989). The relationships between emotion, appraisal, and emotional action readiness. *Journal of Personality and Social Psychology, 57,* 212–228.

Frost, W. D., & Averill, J. R. (1982). Differences between men and women in the everyday experience of anger. In J. R. Averill (Ed.), *Anger and aggression: An essay on emotion* (pp. 281–316). New York: Springer-Verlag.

Fugl-Meyer, A. R., Branholm, I. B., & Fugl-Meyer, K. S. (1991). Happiness and domain-specific life satisfaction in adult Northern Swedes. *Clinical Rehabilitation, 5*(1), 25–33.

Fujita, F., Diener, E., & Sandvik, E. (1991). Gender differences in negative affect and well-being: The case for emotional intensity. *Journal of Personality and Social Psychology, 61*(3), 427–434.

Ganong, L. H., & Coleman, M. (1992). Gender differences in expectations of self and future partner. *Journal of Family Issues, 13*(1), 55–64.

Gayle, B. M., Preiss, R., & Allen, M. (1994). Gender differences and use of conflict strategies. In L. Turner & H. Sterk (Eds.), *Differences that make a difference: Examining assumptions in gender research* (pp. 13–26). Westport, CT: Bergin & Garvey.

Geis, F. L. (1993). Self-fulfilling prophecies: A social psychological view of gender. In A. E. Beall & R. J. Sternberg (Eds.), *The psychology of gender* (pp. 9–54). New York: Guilford Press.

Gershuny, J., & Robinson, J. P. (1988). Historical changes in the household division of labor. *Demography, 25,* 537–552.

Gilbert, L. A. (1993). *Two careers/one family: The promise of gender equality.* Newbury Park, CA: Sage.

Giles, H., & Coupland, (1991). *Language, contexts, and consequences.* Pacific Grove, CA: Brooks/Cole.

Glass, S. P., & Wright, T. L. (1992). Justifications for extramarital relationships: The association between attitudes, behaviors, and gender. *Journal of Sex Research, 29*(3), 361–387.

Gleick, E. (1997). Tower of psychobabble. *Time, 149,* 69–70, 72.

Goetting, A. (1986). Parental satisfaction: A review of research. *Journal of Family Issues, 7,* 83–109.

Goldscheider, F. K., & Waite, L. J. (1991). *New families/no families.* Berkeley: University of California Press.

Goodchilds, J. D., & Zellman, G. L. (1984). Sexual signaling and sexual aggression in adolescent relationships. In N. M. Malamuth & E. Donnerstein (Eds.), *Pornography and sexual aggression* (pp. 233–243). Orlando, FL: Academic Press.

Gottman, J. M. (1979). *Marital interaction: Experimental investigations.* New York: Academic Press.

Gottman, J. M. (1994). *What predicts divorce?* Hillsdale, NJ: Erlbaum.

Gottman, J. M., & Carrere, S. (1994). Why can't men and women get along? Developmental roots and marital inequities. In D. J. Canary & L. Stafford (Eds.), *Communication and relational maintenance* (pp. 203–229). San Diego: Academic Press.

Gottman, J. M., & Krokoff, L. J. (1989). Marital interaction and marital satisfaction: A longitudinal view. *Journal of Consulting and Clinical Psychology, 57,* 47–52.

Gottman, J. M., & Levenson, R. W. (1988). The social psychophysiology of marriage. In P. Noller & M. A. Fitzpatrick (Eds.), *Perspectives on marital interaction* (pp. 182–200). Philadelphia: Multilingual Matters.

Gottman, J. M., & Levenson, R. W. (1992). Marital processes predictive of later dissolution: Behavior, physiology, and health. *Journal of Personality and Social Psychology, 63*(2), 221–233.

Grauerholz, E., & Serpe, R. T. (1985). Initiation and response: The dynamics of sexual interaction. *Sex Roles, 12*(9–10), 1041–1059.

Gray, J. (1992). *Men are from Mars, women are from Venus.* New York: Harper Collins.

Guerrero, L. K., & Andersen, P. A. (1991). The waxing and waning of relational intimacy: Touch as a function of relational stage, gender, and touch avoidance. *Journal of Social and Personal Relationships, 8,* 147–165.

Haas, L. (1982). Determinants of role-sharing behavior: A study of egalitarian couples. *Sex Roles, 8,* 747–760.

Hacker, W. (1985). Activity: A fruitful concept in industrial psychology. In M. Frese & J. Sabini (Eds.), *Goal directed behavior: The concept of action in psychology* (pp. 262–283). Hillsdale, NJ: Erlbaum.

Hall, J. A. (1984). *Nonverbal sex differences: Communication accuracy and expressive style.* Baltimore: Johns Hopkins University Press.

Hall, J. A. (in press). How big are nonverbal sex differences? The case of smiling and sensitivity to nonverbal cues. In D. J. Canary & K. Dindia (Eds.), *Sex differences in communication.* Mahwah, NJ: Erlbaum.

Hall, J. A., & Veccia, E. M. (1990). More "touching" observations: New insights on men, women, and interpersonal touch. *Journal of Personality and Social Psychology, 59,* 1155–1162.

Hammersla, J. F., & Frease-McMahan, L. (1990). University students' priorities: Life goals vs. relationships. *Sex Roles, 23*(1–2), 1–14.

Hare-Mustin, R. T., & Marecek, J. (1988). The meaning of difference: Gender theory, postmodernism, and psychology. *American Psychologist, 43,* 455–464.

Hatfield, E. (1983). What do men and women want from love and sex? In E. R. Allgeier & N. B. McCormick (Eds.), *Changing boundaries: Gender roles and sexual behavior* (pp. 106–134). Palo Alto, CA: Mayfield.

Hatfield, E. (1984). The dangers of intimacy. In V. J. Derlega (Ed.), *Communication, intimacy, and close relationships* (pp. 207–220). Orlando, FL: Academic Press.

Hatfield, E., Sprecher, S., Pillemer, J. T., Greenberger, D., & Wexler, P. (1988). Gender differences in what is desired in the sexual relationship. *Journal of Psychology and Human Sexuality, 1,* 39–52.

Heavey, C. L., Layne, C., & Christensen, A. (1993). Gender and conflict structure in marital interaction: A replication and extension. *Journal of Consulting and Clinical Psychology, 61,* 16–27.

Hecht, M. L., Marston, P. J., & Larkey, L. K. (1994). Love ways and relationship quality in heterosexual relationships. *Journal of Social and Personal Relationships, 11,* 25–43.

Heiss, J. (1991). Gender and romantic-love roles. *Sociological Quarterly, 32,* 575–591.

Helgeson, V. S., Shaver, P., & Dyer, M. (1987). Prototypes of intimacy and distance in same-sex and opposite-sex relationships. *Journal of Social and Personal Relationships, 4,* 195–233.

Hendrick, C., & Hendrick, S. (1991). Dimensions of love: A sociobiological interpretation. *Journal of Social and Clinical Psychology, 10*(2), 206–230.

Hendrick, S. S., & Hendrick, C. (1995). Gender differences and similarities in sex and love. *Personal Relationships, 2*(1), 55–65.

Henley, N. (1977). *Body politics: Power, sex, and non-verbal communication.* Englewood Cliffs, NJ: Prentice-Hall

Heslin, R., & Alper, T. (1983). Touch: A bonding gesture. In J. M. Wiemann & R. Harrison (Eds.), *Nonverbal interaction* (pp. 47–75). Newbury Park, CA: Sage.

Heslin, R., & Boss, D. (1980). Nonverbal intimacy in airport arrival and departure. *Personality and Social Psychology Bulletin, 6,* 248–242.

Heslin, R., Nguyen, T. D., & Nguyen, M. L. (1983). Meanings of touch: The case of touch from a stranger or a same-sex person. *Journal of Nonverbal Behavior, 7,* 147–157.

Hill, C. T., & Stull, D. E. (1987). Gender and self-disclosure: Strategies for exploring the issues. In V. J. Derlega & J. H. Berg (Eds.), *Self-disclosure: Theory, research, and therapy* (pp. 81–100). New York: Plenum Press.

Hiller, D. V. (1984). Power dependence and division of family work. *Sex Roles, 10,* 1003–1019.

Hilton, J. M., & Haldeman, V. A. (1991). Gender differences in the performance of household tasks by adults and children in single-parent and two-parent, two-earner families. *Journal of Family Issues, 12,* 114–130.

Hinde, R. A. (1976). On describing relationships. *Journal of Child Psychology and Psychiatry, 17,* 1–19.

Hite, S. (1987). *Women and love: A cultural revolution in progress.* New York: Knopf.

Hochschild, A. with Machung, A. (1989). *The second shift: Working parents and the revolution at home.* New York: Viking Press.

Holman, T. L., & Jacquart, M. (1988). Leisure-activity patterns and marital satisfaction: A further test. *Journal of Marriage and the Family, 50,* 69–77.

Howard, J. A., Blumstein, P., & Schwartz, P. (1986). Sex, power, and influence tactics in intimate relationships. *Journal of Personality and Social Psychology, 51,* 102–109.

Huber, J., & Spitze, G. (1983). *Sex stratification: Children, housework, and jobs.* New York: Academic Press.

Hyde, J. S., & Linn, M. C. (1988). Gender differences in verbal ability: A meta-analysis. *Psychological Bulletin, 104,* 53–69.

Hyde, J. S., & Plant, E. A. (1995). Magnitude of psychological gender differences: Another side to the story. *American Psychologist, 50,* 159–161.

Ickes, W. (1993). Traditional gender roles: Do they make, and then break, our relationships? *Journal of Social Issues, 49,* 71–83.

Inglis, A., & Greenglass, E. R. (1989). Motivation for marriage among women and men. *Psychological Reports, 65,* 1035–1042.

Inman, C. (1996). Friendships among men: Closeness in the doing. In J. T. Wood (Ed.), *Gendered relationships* (pp. 95–110). Mountain View, CA: Mayfield.

Instone, D., Major, B., & Bunker, B. B. (1983). Gender, self confidence, and social influence strategies: An organizational simulation. *Journal of Personality and Social Psychology, 44,* 322–333.

Izard, C. E. (1991). *The psychology of emotions.* New York: Plenum Press.

James, D., & Clarke, S. (1993). Women, men, and interruptions. In D. Tannen (Ed.), *Gender and conversational interaction* (pp. 231–280). New York: Oxford University Press.

Janisse, M. P., Edguer, N., & Dyck, D. G. (1986). Type A behavior, anger expression, and reactions to anger imagery. *Motivation and Emotion, 10*(4), 371–386.

John, D., Shelton, B. A., & Luschen, K. (1995). Race, ethnicity, gender, and perceptions of fairness. *Journal of Family Issues, 16,* 357–379.

Johnson, F. L. (1996). Friendships among women: Closeness in dialogue. In J. T. Wood (Ed.), *Gendered relationships* (pp. 79–94). Mountain View, CA: Mayfield.

Johnson, F. L., & Aries, E. J. (1983a). Conversational patterns among same-sex pairs of late-adolescent close friends. *Journal of Genetic Psychology, 142,* 225–238.

Johnson, F. L., & Aries, E. J. (1983b). The talk of women friends. *Women's Studies International Forum, 6,* 353–361.

Johnson, K., & Edwards, R. (1991). The effects of gender and type of romantic touch on perceptions of relational commitment. *Journal of Nonverbal Behavior, 15,* 43–55.

Jones, D. C. (1991). Friendship satisfaction and gender: An examination of sex differences in contributors to friendship satisfaction. *Journal of Social and Personal Relationships, 8,* 167–185.

Jones, D. C., Bloys, N., & Wood, M. (1990). Sex roles and friendship patterns. *Sex Roles, 23,* 133–145.

Jones, G. P., & Dembo, M. H. (1989). Age and sex role differences in intimate friendships during childhood and adolescence. *Merrill-Palmer Quarterly, 35,* 445–462.

Jones, S. E. (1986). Sex differences in touch communication. *Western Journal of Speech Communication, 50,* 227–241.

Jourard, S. M. (1966). An exploratory study of body accessibility. *British Journal of Social and Clinical Psychology, 5,* 221–231.

Kalbfleisch, P., & Cody, M. J. (Eds.). (1995). *Gender power, and communication in human relationships.* Hillsdale, NJ: Erlbaum.

Kane, E. (1992). Race, gender, and attitudes toward gender stratification. *Social Psychological Quarterly, 55,* 311–320.

Kane, E. W., & Sanchez, L. (1994). Family status and criticism of gender inequality at home and at work. *Social Forces, 72,* 1079–1102.

Kelley, H. H. (1979). *Personal relationships: Their structure and processes.* Hillsdale, NJ: Erlbaum.

Kenrick, D. T., & Trost, M. R. (1997). Evolutionary approaches to relationships. In S. Duck (Ed.), *Handbook of personal relationships* (pp. 151–177). West Sussex, UK: Wiley.

Kippax, S., Crawford, J., Benton, P., Gault, U., & Noesjirwan, J. (1988). Constructing emotions: Weaving meaning from memories. *British Journal of Social Psychology, 27,* 19–33.

Kippley, J. F. (1994). *Marriage is for keeps: Foundations for Christian marriage.* Cincinnati: Foundation for the Family.

Kleintob, N. A., & Smith, D. A. (1996). Demand–withdraw communication in marital interaction: Tests of interspousal contingency and gender role hypotheses. *Journal of Marriage and the Family, 58,* 945–957.

Kollack, P., Blumstein, P., & Schwartz, P. (1985). Sex and power in interaction: Conversational privileges and duties. *American Sociological Review, 50,* 34–60.

Krokoff, L. J., Gottman, J. M., & Roy, A. K. (1988). Blue-collar and white-collar martial interaction and communication orientation. *Journal of Social and Personal Relationships, 5,* 201–221.

La Gaipa, J. J. (1979). A developmental study of the meaning of friendship in adolescence. *Journal of Adolescence, 2,* 201–213.

Leary, T. (1957). *Interpersonal diagnosis of personality: A functional theory and methodology for personality evaluation.* New York: Ronald Press.

Lee, J. A. (1974, October). The styles of loving. *Psychology Today,* pp. 43–51.

Levenson, R. W., Carstensen, L. L., & Gottman, J. M. (1994). The influence of age and gender on affect, physiology, and their interrelations: A study of long-term marriages. *Journal of Personality and Social Psychology, 67,* 56–68.

Levenson, R. W., Ekman, P., & Friesen, W. V. (1990). Voluntary facial action generates emotion-specific autonomic nervous system activity. *Psychophysiology, 27*(4), 363–384.

Levenson, R. W., & Gottman, J. M. (1983). Marital interaction: Physiological linkage and affective exchange. *Journal of Personality and Social Psychology, 45,* 587–597.

Levenson, R. W., & Gottman, J. M. (1985). Physiological and affective predictors of change in relationship satisfaction. *Journal of Personality and Social Psychology, 49,* 85–94.

Lewis, R. A. (1978). Emotional intimacy among men. *Journal of Social Issues, 34,* 108–121.

Lohr, J. M., Hamberger, L. K., & Bonge, D. (1988). The relationship of factorally validated measures of anger-proneness and irrational beliefs. *Motivation and Emotion, 12*(2), 171–183.

Maccoby, E. E. (1988). Gender as a social category. *Developmental Psychology, 24* 755–765.

Maccoby, E. E. (1990). Gender and relationships: A developmental account. *American Psychologist, 45,* 513–520.

Maccoby, E. E., & Jacklin, C. N. (1974). *The psychology of sex difference.* Stanford, CA: Stanford University Press.

Major, B. (1989). Gender differences in comparisons and entitlement: Implications for comparable worth. *Journal of Social Issues, 45,* 99–115.

Major, B. (1993). Gender, entitlement, and the distribution of family labor. *Journal of Social Issues, 49,* 141–149.

Malos, E. (1995). *The politics of housework.* Cheltenham, UK: New Clarion Press.

Maltz, D. N., & Borker, R. (1982). A cultural approach to male–female miscommunication. In J. Gumperz (Ed.), *Language and social identity* (pp. 196–216). Cambridge, UK: Cambridge University Press.

Manke, B., Seery, B. L., Crouter, A. C., & McHale, S. M. (1994). The three corners of domestic labor: Mothers, fathers, and children's weekday and weekend housework. *Journal of Marriage and the Family, 56,* 657–668.

Marecek, J. (1995). Gender, politics, and psychology's ways of knowing. *American Psychologist, 50,* 162–163.

Maret, E., & Finlay, B. (1984). The distribution of labor among women in dual-earner families. *Journal of Marriage and the Family, 46,* 357–364.

Margolin, G., & Wampold, B. E. (1981). Sequential analysis of conflict and accord in distressed and nondistressed marital partners. *Journal of Consulting and Clinical Psychology, 49,* 554–567.

Margolin, L. (1989). Gender and the prerogatives of dating and marriage: An experimental assessment of a sample of college students. *Sex Roles, 20*(1–2), 91–102.

Markman, H. J., & Notarius, C. L. (1987). Coding marital and family interaction: Current status. In T. Jacob (Ed.), *Family interaction and psychopathology: Theories, methods, and findings* (pp. 329–390). New York: Plenum Press.

Markman, H. J., Silvern, L., Clements, M., & Kraft-Hanak, S. (1993). Men and women dealing with conflict in heterosexual relationships. *Journal of Social Issues, 49,* 107–125.

Marshall, L. L. (1994). Physical and psychological abuse. In W. R. Cupach & B. H. Spitzberg (Eds.), *The dark side of interpersonal communication* (pp. 281–311). Hillsdale, NJ: Erlbaum.

Matula, K. E., Huston, T. L., Grotevant, H. D., & Zamutt, A. (1992). Identity and dating commitment among women and men in college. *Journal of Youth and Adolescence, 21,* 339–356.

McDonald, G. W. (1980). Family power: The assessment of a decade of theory and research, 1970–1979. *Journal of Marriage and the Family, 42,* 841–854.

McPhee, R. D., & Corman, S. R. (1995). An activity-based theory of communication networks in organizations, applied to the case of a local church. *Communication Monographs, 62,* 132–151.

Messman, S. J., Canary, D. J., & Hause, K. S. (1994, February). *Motives, strategies, and equity in the maintenance of opposite-sex friendships.* Paper presented at the Western States Communication Association Convention, San Jose, CA.

Metts, S., & Bowers, J. W. (1994). Emotion in interpersonal communication. In. M. L. Knapp & G. R. Miller (Eds.), *Handbook of interpersonal communication* (2nd ed., pp. 508–541). Thousand Oaks, CA: Sage.

Miller, R. S., & Lefcourt, H. M. (1982). The assessment of social intimacy. *Journal of Personality Assessment, 46,* 514–518.

Monsour, M. (1992). Meanings of intimacy in cross- and same-sex friendships. *Journal of Social and Personal Relationships, 9,* 277–295.

Montgomery, B. M. (1987). *Sexual versus friendly flirting.* Paper presented at the annual conference of the International Communication Association, Montreal, Canada.

Moore, H. L. (1994). Understanding sex and gender. In T. Ingold (Ed.), *Companion encyclopedia of anthropology* (pp. 813–830). New York: Routledge.

Morawski, J. G. (1987). The troubled quest for masculinity, femininity, and androgyny. In P. Shaver & C. Hendrick (Eds.), *Sex and gender* (pp. 44–69). Newbury Park, CA: Sage.

Morton, T. C., Alexander, J. F., & Altman, I. (1976). Communication and relationship definition. In G. R. Miller (Ed.), *Explorations in interpersonal communication* (pp. 105–126). Beverly Hills, CA: Sage.

Mulac, A., & Bradac, J. J. (1995). Women's style in problem solving interaction: Powerless, or simply feminine? In P. J. Kalbfleisch & M. J. Cody (Eds.), *Gender, power, and communication in human relationships* (pp. 83–104). Hillsdale, NJ: Erlbaum.

Narus, L. R., & Fischer, J. L. (1982). Strong but not silent: A re-examination of expressivity in the relationships of men. *Sex Roles, 8*(2), 159–168.

Nicholson, J. (1993). *Men and women: How different are they?* Oxford, UK: Oxford University Press.

Nin, A. (1992). Eroticism in women. In D. Steinberg (Ed.), *The erotic impulse: Honoring the sensual self* (pp. 117–123). New York: Tarcher/Perigee Books.

Noller, P. (1982). Channel consistency and inconsistency in the communications of married couples. *Journal of Personality and Social Psychology, 43,* 732–741.

Noller, P., Feeney, J. A., Bonnell, D., & Callan, V. J. (1994). A longitudinal study of conflict in early marriage. *Journal of Social and Personal Relationships, 11,* 233–252.

Noseworthy, C. M., & Lott, A. J. (1984). The cognitive organization of gender-stereotypic categories. *Personality and Social Psychology Bulletin, 10,* 474–481.

Novaco, R. W. (1975). *Anger control: The development and evaluation of an experimental treatment.* Lexington, MA: Lexington Books.

Oliver, M. B., & Sedikides, C. (1992). Effects of sexual permissiveness on desirability of partner as a function of low and high commitment to relationship. *Social Psychology Quarterly, 55,* 321–333.

Orthner, D. K. (1985). Conflict and leisure interaction in families. In R. G. Gunter, J. Stanley, & R. St. Clair (Eds.), *Transitions to leisure: Conceptual and human issues* (pp. 133–139). Lanham, MD: University Press of America.

Pearson, J. C., Turner, L. H., & Mancillas, W. T. (1991). *Gender and communication.* Dubuque, IA: William C. Brown.

Perlman, D., & Fehr, B. (1987). The development of intimate relationships. In D. Perlman & S. Duck (Eds.), *Intimate relationships: Development, dynamics, and deterioration* (pp. 13–42). Newbury Park, CA: Sage.

Perper, T. (1985). *Sex signals: The biology of love.* Philadelphia: ISI Press.

Pervin, L. A. (1986). Personal and social determinants of behavior in situations. In A. Furham (Ed.), *Social behavior in context* (pp. 81–102). Boston: Allyn & Bacon.

Planalp, S. (1992, November). *Cognition and/or emotion in close relationships.* Paper presented at the Speech Communication Association Convention, Chicago, IL.

Pleck, J. H. (1977). The work–family role system. *Social Problems, 24,* 417–427.

Pleck, J. H. (1985). *Working wives/working husbands.* Beverly Hills, CA: Sage.

Prager, K. J. (1989). Intimacy status and couple communication. *Journal of Social and Personal Relationships, 6,* 435–449.

Prager, K. J. (1995). *The psychology of intimacy.* New York: Boston: Allyn & Bacon.

Putnam, L. L. (1982). In search of gender: A critique of communication and sex roles research. *Women's Studies in Communication, 5,* 1–9.

Putnam, L. L., & Wilson, C. E. (1982). Communication strategies in organizational conflict: Reliability and validity of a measurement scale. In M. Burgoon (Ed.), *Communication yearbook 6* (pp. 629–652). Beverly Hills, CA: Sage.

Quackenbush, R. L. (1990). Sex roles and social-sexual effectiveness. *Social Behavior and Personality, 18,* 35–39.

Radley, A. (1988). The social form of feeling. *British Journal of Social Psychology, 27,* 5–18.

Ragan, S. L. (1989). Communication between the sexes: A consideration of differences in adult communication. In J. F. Nussbaum (Ed.), *Life-span communication: Normative processes* (pp. 179–193). Hillsdale, NJ: Erlbaum.

Rakow, L. (1986). Rethinking gender research in communication. *Journal of Communication, 36,* 11–26.

Raush, H. L., Barry, W. A., Hertel, R. J., & Swain, M. A. (1974). *Communication, conflict, and marriage.* San Francisco: Jossey-Bass.

Rawlins, W. K. (1992). *Friendship matters: Communication, dialectics, and the life course.* Hawthorne, NY: Aldine de Gruyter.

Rawlins, W. K. (1993). Communication in cross-sex friendships. In L. P. Arliss & D. Borisoff (Eds.), *Women and men communicating* (pp. 51–70). Fort Worth, TX: Harcourt Brace Jovanovich.

Reis, H. T. (in press). Gender differences in intimacy and related behaviors: Context and process. In D. J. Canary & K. Dindia (Eds.), *Sex differences in communication.* Mahwah, NJ: Erlbaum.

Reis, H. T., Senchak, M., & Solomon, B. (1985). Sex differences in the intimacy of social interaction: Further examination of potential explanations. *Journal of Personality and Social Psychology, 48,* 1204–1217.

Reisman, J. M. (1990). Intimacy in same-sex friendships. *Sex Roles, 23,* 65–82.

Rhode, D. L. (1990). Theoretical perspectives on sexual difference. In D. L. Rhode (Ed.), *Theoretical perspectives on sexual difference* (pp. 1–9). New Haven, CT: Yale University Press.

Robey, E. B., Canary, D. J., & Burggraf, C. S. (in press). Conversational maintenance behaviors of husbands and wives: An observational analysis. In D. J. Canary & K. Dindia (Eds.), *Sex differences in communication.* Mahwah, NJ: Erlbaum.

Robins, C. J. (1986). Sex role perceptions and social anxiety in opposite-sex and same-sex situations. *Sex Roles, 14*(7–8), 383–395.

Robinson, J. P. (1980). Housework technology and household work. In S. F. Berk (Ed.), *Women and household labor* (pp. 53–67). Beverly Hills, CA: Sage.

Rose, S. (1985). Same- and cross-sex friendships and the psychology of homosociality. *Sex Roles, 12*(1), 63–74.

Rosenfeld, L. (1979). Self-disclosure avoidance: Why I am afraid to tell you who I am. *Communication Monographs, 46,* 63–74.

Rosenfeld, L. B., Kartus, S., & Ray, C. (1976). Body accessibility revisited. *Journal of Communication, 26,* 27–30.

Ross, C. E. (1987). The division of labor at home. *Social Forces, 65,* 816–833.

Rotter, N. G., & Rotter, G. S. (1988). Sex differences in the encoding and decoding of negative facial emotions. *Journal of Nonverbal Behavior, 12*(2), 139–148.

Rowe, R., & Snizek, W. E. (1995). Gender differences in work values: Perpetuating the myth. *Work and Occupations, 22,* 215–229.

Rubin, L. B. (1990). *Erotic wars: What happened to the sexual revolution?* New York: Harper Perennial.

Rubin, Z., Peplau, L. A., & Hill, C. T. (1980). Loving and leaving: Sex differences in romantic attachments. *Sex Roles, 6,* 821–835.

Rusbult, C. E. (1987). Responses to dissatisfaction in close relationships: The exit–voice–loyalty–neglect model. In D. Perlman & S. Duck (Eds.), *Intimate relationships: Development, dynamics, and deterioration* (pp. 209–237). Newbury Park, CA: Sage.

Rusbult, C. E., & Buunk, B. P. (1993). Commitment processes in close relationships: An interdependence analysis. *Journal of Social and Personal Relationships, 10,* 175–204.

Rusbult, C. E., Drigotas, S. M., & Verette, J. (1994). The investment model: An interdependence analysis of commitment processes and relationship maintenance phenomena. In D. J. Canary & L. Stafford (Eds.), *Communication and relational maintenance* (pp. 115–139). San Diego: Academic Press.

Rusbult, C. E., Verette, J., Whitney, G. A., Slovik, L. F., & Lipkus, I. (1991). Accommodation processes in close relationships: Theory and preliminary empirical evidence. *Journal of Personality and Social Psychology, 60,* 53–78.

Sagrestano, L. M. (1992). Power strategies in personal relationships. *Psychology of Women Quarterly, 16,* 481–495.

Sagrestano, L. M., Christensen, A., & Heavey, C. L. (in press). Sex differences in managing conflict: The demand-withdrawal pattern. In D. J. Canary & K. Dindia (Eds.), *Sex differences in communication.* Mahwah, NJ: Erlbaum.

Sapadin, L. A. (1988). Friendship and gender: Perspectives of professional men and women. *Journal of Social and Personal Relationships, 5,* 387–403.

Sayers, S. L., & Baucom, D. H. (1991). Role of femininity and masculinity in distressed couples' communication. *Journal of Personality and Social Psychology, 61,* 641–647.

Schaap, C., Buunk, B., & Kerkstra, A. (1988). Marital conflict resolution. In P. Noller & M. A. Fitzpatrick (Eds.), *Perspectives on marital interaction* (pp. 203–244). Philadelphia: Multilingual Matters.

Schaefer, M., & Olson, D. (1981). Assessing intimacy: The PAIR Inventory. *Journal of Marriage and Family Therapy, 7,* 47–60.

Scherer, K. R., & Tannenbaum, P. H. (1986). Emotional experiences in everyday life: A survey approach. *Motivation and Emotion, 10,* 295–314.

Schutz, W. (1967). *The interpersonal underworld: Fundamentals of interpersonal relationship orientation.* Palo Alto, CA: Science and Behavior Books.

Scott, J. W. (1996). Gender: A useful category of historical analysis. In J. W. Scott (Ed.), *Feminism and history* (pp. 152–180). New York: Oxford University Press.

Shaver P., & Hendrick, C. (Eds.). (1987). *Sex and gender.* Newbury Park, CA: Sage.

Shaver, P., Schwartz, J., Kirson, D., & O'Connor, C. (1987). Emotion knowledge: Further exploration of a prototypic approach. *Journal of Personality and Social Psychology, 52*(6), 1061–1086.

Shaw, S. M. (1985). Gender and leisure: Inequality in the distribution of leisure time. *Journal of Leisure Research, 17,* 266–282.

Shaw, S. M. (1993). Dereifying family leisure: An examination of women's and men's everyday experiences and perceptions of family time. *Leisure Studies, 14,* 271–286.

Shelton, B. A. (1990). The distribution of household tasks: Does wife's employment status make a difference? *Journal of Family Issues, 11,* 115–135.

Shelton, B. A. (1992). *Women, men, and time: Gender differences in paid work, housework, and leisure.* New York: Greenwood Press.

Sheinberg, M., & Penn., P. (1991). Gender dilemmas, gender questions, and the gender mantra. *Journal of Marital and Family Therapy, 17,* 33–44.

Sherman, M. D., & Thelen, M. H. (1996). Fear of Intimacy Scale: Validation and extension with adolescents. *Journal of Social and Personal Relationships, 13,* 507–521.

Siegman, A. W. (1994). Cardiovascular consequences of expressing and repressing anger. In A. W. Siegman & T. W. Smith (Eds.), *Anger, hostility, and the heart* (pp. 173–197). Hillsdale, NJ: Erlbaum.

Sillars, A. L., & Wilmot, W. W. (1994). Communication strategies in conflict and mediation. In J. A. Daly & J. M. Wiemann (Eds.), *Strategic interpersonal communication* (pp. 163–190). Hillsdale, NJ: Erlbaum.

Silver, H., & Goldscheider, F. (1994). Flexible work and housework: Work and family constraints on women's domestic labor. *Social Forces, 72,* 1103–1119.

Six, B., & Eckles, T. (1991). A closer look at the complex structure of gender stereotypes. *Sex Roles, 24,* 57–71.

Smith, G. T., Snyder, D. K., Trull, T. J., & Monsma, B. R. (1988). Predicting relationship satisfaction from couples' use of leisure time. *American Journal of Family Therapy, 16* 3–13.

Smuts, B. (1995). The evolutionary origins of patriarchy. *Human Nature, 6,* 1–32.

Snell, W. E. (1989). Willingness to self-disclose to female and male friends as a function of social anxiety and gender. *Personality and Social Psychology Bulletin, 15,* 113–125.

Snyder, M. (1987). *Public appearances/private realities: The psychology of self-monitoring.* New York: W. H. Freeman.

Sollie, D. L., & Fischer, J. L. (1985). Sex-role orientation, intimacy of topic, and target person differences in self-disclosure among women. *Sex Roles, 12,* 917–929.

South, S. J., & Spitze, G. (1994). Housework in marital and nonmarital households. *American Sociological Review, 59,* 327–347.

Spence, J. T., Helmreich, R. L., & Stapp, J. (1974). The Personal Attributes Questionnaire: A measure of sex-role stereotypes and masculinity–femininity. *JSAS Catalog of Selected Documents in Psychology, 4,* 43–44.

Spitzberg, B. H. (1997). Violence in intimate relationships. In W. R. Cupach & D. J. Canary (Eds.), *Competence in interpersonal conflict* (pp. 175–201). New York: McGraw-Hill.

Spitze, G. (1988). Women's employment and family relations: A review. *Journal of Marriage and the Family, 50,* 595–618.

Sprecher, S. (1985). Sex differences in bases of power in dating relationships. *Sex Roles, 12,* 449–462.

Sprecher, S. (1986). The relationship between inequity and emotions in close relationships. *Social Psychological Quarterly, 49,* 309–321.

Sprecher, S., & McKinney, K. (1993). *Sexuality.* Newbury Park, CA: Sage.

Stafford, L., & Canary, D. J. (1991). Maintenance strategies and romantic relationship type, gender, and relational characteristics. *Journal of Social and Personal Relationships, 8,* 217–242.

Stafford, M. C., & Galle, O. G. (1984). Victimization rates, exposure to risk, and fear of crime. *Criminology, 22,* 173–185.

Stafford, L., & Reske, J. (1990). Idealization and communication in long-distance premarital relationships. *Family Relations, 39,* 274–279.

Stamp, G. H. (1994). The appropriation of the parental role through communication during the transition to parenthood. *Communication Monographs, 61,* 89–112.

Statham, A. (1987). The gender model revisited: Difference in the management styles of men and women. *Sex Roles, 16,* 409–429

Steinberg, L. (1981). Transformations in family relations at puberty. *Developmental Psychology, 17,* 833–840.

Steinberg, L. D., & Hill, J. P. (1978). Patterns of family interaction as a function of age, the onset of puberty, and formal thinking. *Developmental Psychology, 14,* 683–684.

Stets, J. E. (1993). Control in dating relationships. *Journal of Marriage and the Family, 55,* 673–685.

Strasser, S. M. (1980). An enlarged human existence? Technology and household work in nineteenth-century America. In S. F. Berk (Ed.), *Women and household labor* (pp. 29–51). Beverly Hills, CA: Sage.

Street, R. L., & Murphy, T. L. (1987). Interpersonal orientation and speech behavior. *Communication Monographs, 54,* 42–62.

Strodbeck, F. L., & Mann, R. D. (1956). Sex role differentiation in jury deliberations. *Sociometry, 19,* 3–11.

Swain, S. (1989). Covert intimacy: Closeness in men's friendships. In B. J.

Riseman & P. Schwartz (Eds.), *Gender in intimate relationships* (pp. 71–86). Belmont, CA: Wadsworth.

Swim, J., Borgida, E., Maruyama, G., & Meyers, D. G. (1989). Joan McKay versus John McKay: Do gender stereotypes bias evaluations? *Psychological Bulletin, 105,* 409–429.

Tannen, D. (1990). *You just don't understand: Women and men in conversation.* New York: William Morrow.

Tannen, D. (Ed.). (1993). *Gender and conversational interaction.* New York: Oxford University Press.

Tannen, D. (1994). *Gender and discourse.* New York: Oxford University Press.

Thompson, L. (1991). Family work: Women's sense of fairness. *Journal of Family Issues, 12,* 181–196.

Thompson, L., & Walker, A. J. (1989). Gender in families. *Journal of Marriage and the Family, 51,* 845–871.

Thorne, B. (1990). Children and gender: Construction of difference. In D. L. Rhode (Ed.), *Theoretical perspectives on sexual difference* (pp. 100–113). New Haven, CT: Yale University Press.

Thorne, B., Kramarae, C., & Henley, N. (Eds.) (1983). *Language, gender, and society* (2nd ed.). Rowley, MA: Newbury House.

Tiefer, L. (1995). *Sex is not a natural act and other essays.* Boulder, CO: Westview Press.

Ting-Toomey, S. (1983). An analysis of verbal communication patterns in high and low marital adjustment groups. *Human Communication Research, 9,* 306–319.

Ting-Toomey, S. (1991). Intimacy expressions in three cultures: France, Japan, and the United States. *International Journal of Intercultural Relations, 15*(1), 29–46.

Tompkins, S. S. (1962). *Affect, imagery, and consciousness: Vol. 1. The positive effects.* New York: Springer-Verlag.

Tompkins, S. S. (1963). *Affect, imagery, and consciousness: Vol. 2. The negative effects.* New York: Springer-Verlag.

Toner, H. L., & Gates, G. R. (1985). Emotional traits and recognition of facial expression of emotion. *Journal of Nonverbal Behavior, 9*(1), 48–66.

Townsend, J. M. (1995). Sex without emotional involvement: An evolutionary interpretation of sex differences. *Archives of Sexual Behavior, 24,* 173–206.

Trost, M. R., & Alberts, J. K. (in press). An evolutionary view of understanding gender effects in communicating attraction. In D. J. Canary & K. Dindia (Eds.), *Sex, gender, and communication: Similarities and differences.* Mahwah, NJ: Erlbaum.

Tschann, J. M. (1988). Self-disclosure in adult friendship: Gender and marital status differences. *Journal of Social and Personal Relationships, 5,* 65–81.

Turner, H. A. (1994). Gender and social support: Taking the bad with the good? *Sex Roles, 30*(7–8), 521–541.

van de Vliert, E., & Euwema, M. C. (1994). Agreeableness and activeness as components of conflict behaviors. *Journal of Personality and Social Psychology, 66,* 674–687.

Vangelisti, A. (1994). Messages that hurt. In W. R. Cupach & B. H. Spitzberg (Eds.), *The dark side of interpersonal communication* (pp. 53–82). Hillsdale, NJ: Erlbaum.

Van Yperen, N. W., & Buunk, B. P. (1990). A longitudinal study of equity and satisfaction in intimate relationships. *European Journal of Social Psychology, 20,* 287–309.

Vaughter, R. M., Sadh, D., & Vozzola, E. (1994). Sex similarities and differences in types of play in games and sports. *Psychology of Women Quarterly, 18,* 85–104.

Waldron, V., & Di Mare, L. (in press). Gender as a culturally determined construct: Communication styles in Japan and the United States. In D. J. Canary & K. Dindia (Eds.), *Sex differences in communication.* Mahwah, NJ: Erlbaum.

Warr, M. (1984). Fear of victimization: Why are women and the elderly more afraid? *Social Science Quarterly, 65,* 681–702.

Warr, M. (1992). Altruistic fear of victimization in households. *Social Science Quarterly, 73*(4), 723–736.

Wessman, A. E., & Ricks, J. H. (1966). *Mood and personality.* New York: Holt, Rinehart & Winston.

White, L. K., & Brinkerhoff, D. B. (1981). Children's work in the family: Its significance and meaning. *Journal of Marriage and the Family, 43,* 789–798.

Wilkins, B. M., & Andersen, P. A. (1991). Gender differences and similarities in management communication: A meta-analysis. *Management Communication Quarterly, 5,* 6–35.

Wilson, M. N. (1986). Perceived parental activity of mothers, fathers, and grandmothers in three generational black families. *Journal of Black Psychology, 12,* 43–60.

Wilson, M. N., Tolson, T. F. J., Hinton, I. D., & Kiernan, M. (1990). Flexibility and sharing of child care duties in black families. *Sex Roles, 22,* 409–425.

Wong, H. (1981). Typologies of intimacy. *Psychology of Women Quarterly, 5*(3), 435–443.

Wood, J. T. (1993). Engendered relations: Interaction, caring, power, and responsibility in intimacy. In S. Duck (Ed.), *Social context and relationships* (pp. 26–55). Thousand Oaks, CA: Sage.

Wood, J. T. (1996). *Gendered relationships.* Mountain View, CA: Mayfield.

Wood, J. T., & Dindia, K. (in press). What is the difference? A dialogue about differences and similarities between women and men. In D. J. Canary & K. Dindia (Eds.), *Sex differences in communication.* Mahwah, NJ: Erlbaum.

Wood, W. (1987). Meta-analytic review of sex differences in group performance. *Psychological Bulletin, 102,* 53–71.

Wood, W., & Karten, S. J. (1986). Sex differences in interaction style as a product of perceived sex differences in competence. *Journal of Personality and Social Psychology, 50,* 341–347.

Wood, W., Rhodes, N., & Whelan, M. (1989). Sex differences in positive well-being: A consideration of emotional style and marital status. *Psychological Bulletin, 106*(2), 249–264.

Wright, P. H. (in press). Toward an expanded orientation to the study of sex differences in friendship. In D. J. Canary & K. Dindia (Eds.), *Sex differences in communication.* Mahwah, NJ: Erlbaum.

Zietlow, P. H., & Sillars, A. L. (1988). Life stage differences in communication during marital conflicts. *Journal of Social and Personal Relationships, 5,* 223–245.

Zillmann, D. (1990). The interplay of cognition and excitation in aggravated conflict among intimates. In D. D. Cahn (Ed.), *Intimates in conflict: A communication perspective* (pp. 187–208). Hillsdale, NJ: Erlbaum.

Zimmerman, D. H., & West, C. (1975). Sex roles, interruptions, and silences in conversations. In B. Thorne & N. Henley (Eds.), *Language and sex: Differences and dominance* (pp. 105–129). Rowley, MA: Newbury House.

Zuckerman, D. M. (1989). Stress, self-esteem, and mental health: How does gender make a difference? *Sex Roles, 20*(7–8), 429–444.

Index